six until me

Essays from a life with diabetes

By Kerri Sparling

Dedication

For Chris, because it was all his idea

Introduction

Growing Up with Diabetes

Urine Charge with the Pee Alarm
Postcards from Eddie
Kitty
Memories
"You said the esh word."
Stings
Click, Clack, Click, Clack
Diaries of a Diabetic Girl
What Happened at Lunch ("Sorry, mom.")
The Curse of the Camp Coleslaw
Chopping Broccoli
Between Dinner and a Movie
More Than Candy and Costumes
Your Mama is so Awesome
What Helped Me as a Kid with Diabetes
Twenty-Five Years with Diabetes: What I've Learned
Thirty-One Years with Diabetes
A Letter to a Younger Me

Diabetes in the Wild

The Droid You're Looking For
PWD in the Wild
Insulin Pump on the Beach
The Friendly Skies
McDave from the Plane
We Made Contact
Overnight Flight
So Much Bigger
Airport Connections
Close, But(t) Not Close Enough
America Runs on Insulin
"Bag got run over."
Pumped for the Pizza Man
Hawkey Playah
The Mothership
These Boots Were Made for Talking

Diabetes Shorthand
Unexpected Advocacy

Diabetes Community

People Who Need People
On Paper
Fine
Advice for Newbies
Twice
The Scaffolding
Diabetes Club
Joslin Medalists
Ordinary but Extraordinary
The Quiet Parts

Mentalbetes

Define or Explain
What's it like to take insulin?
Duck on a Pond
Sick Your Whole Life
Complicated
Progress
Filling Back Up
Change Just One Thing
At Least It's Not
Full Body
The Gray Area
Voicemail for my Pancreas

Healthcare Experiences

Lies
Just a Job
Time Consuming
Trapped by Shipments and Timeouts
How to Improve my Healthcare Experience
A Cleaning
Being a Rotten Patient
Share and Don't Share

Things You Eat and Things that Beep
Crabs
Froast
Grocery Wars
Rocco Returns
Hungry
Someone Else's Childhood
In a Pickle
Diabetes Food Lies
Starting the Pump
"Do you like it?"
Why I Pump
Rage Bolus
Disco Boobs
Toss 'Em in the Big Blue Hole
How to Have Sex with an Insulin Pump

Highs and Lows
A Jacket, Just in Case
Disclosures
Emergency Plan
Employee of the Month
Bullets
Jet-Lagged
Lunchtime Lows
Sad Robot
Seven Versions of a Low Blood Sugar
Cleaning Crews
A Sobering Experience
Evidence
Good Luck, Lady
Low Hangovers
Parking Lot Lows
Whine
Hypo Effery
Pulled Over
Half a Juice Box
Oh, High!

Parenting
Moody, Pregnant Mess
Ignoring Her
Things I Learned in my First Year as a Diabetic Mommy
How I Talk about Diabetes with my Kids
Iron Mom
The Question
For Your Blood's Sugar
Proof in the Pretend Pudding
Put On Your Listening Ears
Instead of Making Insulin
Motherhood with Diabetes
Do You Wish You Didn't Have Diabetes?
A Matter of Apologies
The One About Steel Magnolias
Learning Empathy
Thoughts on Being a Mom with Type 1 Diabetes

Afterword

Glossary

"She Still Smiles"

Disclosures

Acknowledgments

Introduction

Just before second grade, I started to wet the bed again. I seemed healthy, otherwise, so my parents' response to this bedwetting revival was to buy an alarm that connected to my underpants.

"If you start to pee, these two metal pieces will connect and an alarm will go off. That way, you won't wet the bed and you can get up and use the bathroom!" My mom seemed pleased, hoping this would fix the problem.

"Okay," I said. I was embarrassed that I was wetting the bed. I hadn't wet the bed in years. And a pee alarm?! I was mad I couldn't control this; I remember that frustration clearly. I wore the pee alarm for about two weeks, and after waking up almost every night with my underpants going off like a fire engine siren, I was scared but dry.

A week before I was scheduled to start school, my mother took me in for my before-school physical.

"Just wipe with these special wipes – front to back, Kerri – and pee into the cup. Close it up, bring it out, and we'll have everything we need!" The nurse smiled at me while my mother and the pediatrician talked about how excited I was to start school. We were just a few hours away from receiving a phone call that would reshape my world.

I was diagnosed with type 1 diabetes on September 11, 1986. I spent twelve nights in Rhode Island Hospital, learning to give practice injections of saline to an orange.

"We use an orange because its skin is most like human skin," the diabetes educator explained. Which is when it dawned on me that these needles were intended for *my* skin. And at that moment, success was redefined by having the guts to press these needles into my body, every day, for the rest of my life.

The learning curve was steep. My mom learned to give me injections, and she'd press the needle tip against my skin slowly and steadily, aiming with a steady hand, while my father gave my injections like I was a dart board and his challenge was to hit the bullseye as quickly and efficiently as possible.

This was our new normal. Life went on, albeit adjusted.

When I was diagnosed with type 1 diabetes at the age of seven, I didn't feel alone because my family was there with me. We did this as a team. But as I grew up and started to explore a life of my own, I realized I didn't know many adults who also had diabetes.

I didn't have any friends who understood the weird triumph of a soft blood sugar landing after pizza. I didn't know anyone else who had treated a low by having to eat the dirt-covered Swedish Fish candies from the floor mats of the car. I was the only person who was counting carbs and calculating insulin doses.

Everyone I knew made their own insulin. But when I started writing about diabetes online at SixUntilMe.com, I wasn't alone anymore. What I've learned by connecting with the diabetes community has been nothing short of life-saving.

I wrote my first blog post on May 4, 2005 and since that day, I've been immersed in a digital community of people who understand all the nuanced moments of a diabetes life.

At first, my boyfriend read it. And my mom read it. And two of my friends read it. But then two other people found it. And I found a handful of others. And I wasn't alone with diabetes anymore.

The diabetes online community didn't start with blogs. The first mention I found of an online community anchored by diabetes was from UseNet Z*Net International Atari Online Magazine, March 6, 1992, Issue #92-10. David Groves, who had a low blood sugar while driving, wrote about his experience, looking to see if this had happened to others. But the foundation provided by discussion groups and forums is what sites like SixUntilMe.com were built on, and I'm so grateful for the digital storytellers who have come before me.

These essays were once published in a chronological timeline but are now collated by topic. (Which explains why one essay might mention 29 years of diabetes while the next one talks about 33 years of diabetes. Or why my children age un-chronologically. My timelines are unsupervised.) I've included a glossary of terms used and some of the people mentioned, which will hopefully help add some context to this collection of stories, especially if you haven't read SixUntilMe.com in the past. There are disclosures at the end of the book, too; please check those out.

I scroll through the pages of this book, reading some of the older essays, and I'm really proud to be part of a community that shares like this. One that feels like this. One that loves like this. My blog is part of what has become a huge community, where each story about life with diabetes matters, no matter how seemingly small.

I hope you find something here that makes you feel empowered and less alone with diabetes. There is life after diagnosis, and it is filled with hope and possibility.

Thanks for being here.

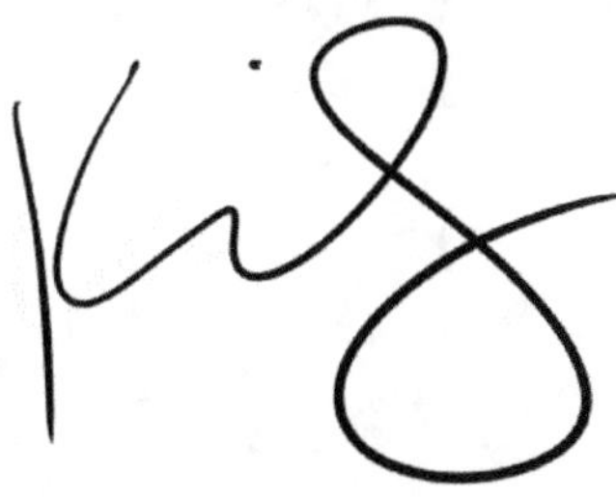

Growing Up
with Diabetes

Growing Up with Diabetes

This year, 2022, marks 36 years with type 1 diabetes. I was diagnosed at the age of seven. When I was diagnosed, the standard of care was to spend a week or two in the hospital, learning how to give insulin injections with orange-capped syringes, test blood sugars, and learn about the best ways to eat with diabetes.

Even though at-home glucose meters were available, I came home from the hospital with a urinalysis kit to check my glucose. It wasn't until a few years ago that I learned my mother actually asked for the urine kit instead of the blood glucose one, because she was overwhelmed by all the elements of diabetes that came flooding into our lives. She needed the opportunity to go slowly as we adjusted to this new life.

Devices like insulin pumps and continuous glucose meters weren't on the market yet. Care was arduous and diabetes management was fragmented. And my parents were scared. (I was scared, too.) We had a lot to learn and we needed to learn it almost instantly. And then we had to figure out life after diagnosis, and remind ourselves how to make that awesome.

I was diagnosed in September, after a visit to the pediatrician. I was picked up early from soccer practice and taken immediately to the hospital.

This first collection of essays focuses on my earlier memories of life with type 1 diabetes.

Urine in Charge with the Pee Alarm

Before I was diagnosed with type 1 diabetes, I started wetting the bed.

We didn't know to check for diabetes. I wasn't exhibiting any other symptoms. But on a somewhat regular basis, my mother was changing my sheets and I was turning my pajamas into soggy bottoms.

"What do we do?"

My parents bought a pee alarm. (You can still buy these things on Amazon, re-marketed as a "Chummie." Memory confirms it was not anyone's chum.) It was this device that included a speaker attached to wires that had metal nodes on the ends of the wires, and you'd clip the two pieces to underpants, one on the inside of the underpants and on one the outside. If you introduced liquid to this environment (aka if you started to pee your pants while sleeping), the two metal nodes would connect and a small electrical currant would course between them, causing an alarm to sound.

And not just any alarm. This alarm was everything current CGM alarms *wished* they could be. It rang out without warning at ten thousand decibels, ripping through ear drums and making the cats all puffed up from fear. The sound would cut through the dead of night, blaring like a siren from my pants, vaulting me out of my bed and tearing down the hallway towards my parents' room, where they'd fumble awkwardly to disconnect the metal nodes.

The noise would bring my four-year-old sister running in from her room, vaulting herself into the middle of my parents' bed. And my brother from his room, karate chopping invisible enemies with his 12-year-old hands.

All while my underpants wailed.

The alarm did its job. Instead of wetting the bed, I woke up several times a night. Later that year, I was diagnosed with type 1 diabetes. The pee alarm was put into a box in the closet.

I do not know who made the initial purchase recommendation, but I do know that my mother kept the pee alarm. And long after my diagnosis, my mother put the alarm in a box and presented it to me as a gift.

Upon opening it, I immediately connected the metal nodes to see if it would still alarm. It did. I laughed for so long and with such horror that I almost needed the alarm again.

Postcards from Eddie

Sometimes the only concrete proof that diabetes hasn't been with me forever are the cards my classmates sent home from school.

Made from manila paper, the kind found in abundance in elementary school, the kids in my class used their Dixon Ticonderoga No. 2 pencils and a fistful of crayons to let me know they were thinking about me.

"Dear Kerri, I heard you were sick. We cleaned out our desks yesterday. You left your lunch here. The pear was all rotten. Hope you feel better soon. – Mike." This card was illustrated in pencil, showing a skeleton picking up a spoiled bag lunch from the garbage can.

"Dear Kerri, Get well soon! Love, Megan." A rainbow of three colors, – pink, blue, and purple – sprawled across the sky, represented by one line. A tree with two apples hanging enormously from its branches stood exactly the same height as the building labeled "Hospitoll."

These cards are safely packed away, somewhere at my dad's house, with the pee alarm and the old blue comfort pillow that I used to clutch while I sucked my thumb. My mother always claimed that she'd give me these things before my wedding day, a promise she followed through on when my husband and I married in 2008.

Even if I never see them again, I remember the cards. I remember snippets of those years like they were postcards from someone else's life.

A picture of the carousel near my childhood home brings back memories of black raspberry ice cream, riding my bike into the beach village with that Jack of Hearts card stuck in the rear tire, and collecting the perfect, miniature shells that washed up on the shoreline after the hurricanes made their rounds.

No memories of a finger stick or an injection. But I do remember that, if I rode my bike all the way to the beach, I could have ice cream without taking an insulin shot.

I don't remember everything about my diagnosis. Doctors spoke mostly to my parents. My dad paced the room and looked out the window. My mom sat at the table with the endocrinologist, listening and taking notes. Books on long and short acting insulin, a regimented diet, and a chart to log my blood sugars slid across the table.

I wasn't paying too much attention to these attempts at education. The 13-year-old boy who shared my hospital room had been bitten by a poisonous spider and was hooked up to an IV drip bag that I found much more interesting. The bite mark was an angry pink and the boy said it itched tremendously.

He and his IV pole and me with my stuffed animal Kitty sat in the children's ward and watched television. He introduced himself as Eddie. I told him my name, too.

"What are you in for?" He raked his fingers down the side of his ankle, where the bite waged a war of infection and venom.

"I have diabetes."

"Oh. I've got a spider bite."

"Wow. Can I see it?"

"Sure." He rolled up his pant leg and exposed the sore. "Where's yours?"

"I don't have any marks on me," I responded. We watched TV while our parents talked to doctors.

In a box in my attic today, I found a postcard from Eddie. We corresponded as pen pals over the course of several years. I remember writing to him about cats and going to the beach, ice cream and bike rides, but never diabetes.

Kitty

They told me I had to go into the hospital for a few weeks. I wasn't exactly sure what "diabetes" meant, but I knew it might involve vampires, because people were drawing my blood every few hours.

"You can pick any friend you'd like to bring with you to the hospital. Any one you want."

My father held my hand as we walked into Ray Willis' Toy Store and I looked at the rows and rows of cuddly and soft stuffed animals. My sneakers scuffed against the tile floor as I examined the options.

The soft ears of a gray elephant looked so nice. I could picture myself hiding behind them if I was scared. I saw an amber-eyed puppy dog with a pokey little nose. He looked like he could be my friend.

Then I saw him.

Kitty.

A huggable, marmalade-colored stuffed animal cat with bright eyes and a long, fluffy tail. He was sandwiched between a giraffe with the tongue sticking out and a stuffed octopus. I reached out and grabbed him from the shelf.

"This one? Is this one okay?"

My father gave me the thumbs up. "That one looks good to me."

Mom and Dad paid for Kitty and we started our drive up to the hospital for my overnight stay. Originally named "Tigger" but eventually falling victim to a less imaginative moniker of "Kitty," I kept this stuffed animal at my side for every blood test and doctor visit. He was a loyal friend and received the occasional shot, too, when I wasn't feeling brave enough to be the only one being injected.

I used to wag his tail and make him wiggle about, trying to convince people in the hospital elevators that he was real.

A boy on the bus in second grade tried to pull Kitty's arm off and gave him a good rip. I cried to my mother, who was about to sew up the wound with orange thread, that she needed to use black thread so it would look like a stitch and I would know he was better. Ever-obliging, my mother stitched Kitty up and I admired his fixable wound with fascination.

Decades later and no longer the newly-diagnosed little girl at the toy store, I've had this Kitty with me through it all. He used to look vibrant and fluffy, but now his fur is matted and mangy. He lived on my bed in college. He moved to my first apartment with me after college. And now he lives in the home where my own children are growing up.

Even when I felt too grown-up to have a stuffed animal on display in my house, Kitty has managed to weasel his way into a bookcase or a closet shelf. Currently, he lives on top of my winter sweaters in my closet, looking at me through his matted fur, with sad eyes from the mountain of wool and cotton.

He made me feel comforted. Admittedly, he still does.

He's a testament to how long it's been. How much I've overcome.

How far I'll go.

Memories

I remember being nine or ten years old, on my hands and knees, crawling up the stairs to get to the kitchen, where my mom was cooking dinner.

I remember calling out for my mom, but the words lost their form and their letters fell into a heap on the staircase.

I remember my mom sitting on the kitchen floor with me, breaking graham crackers into smaller bites and putting them in my mouth, dinner burning in pans on the stove. I remember my mom's eyes being very wide but she wasn't visibly upset. I remember a glass of juice. I remember it was hard to chew because I was crying but I wasn't sure why, and then there's a sharp edit in my memory, where I don't have any recollection of what happened next.

As quickly as it came, the low blood sugar passed. I don't remember what caused it. I don't remember what my face looked like, or how empty my eyes must have been, or what I sounded like as I called for my mom. I don't remember recovering. I don't remember thinking about it for days afterwards. I don't remember feeling affected by it for more than those few minutes.

I see my mother, cleaning up the cracker crumbs and placing the juice glass in the sink, salvaging what was left of the dinner she was cooking, trying to forget.

"You Said the Esh Word."

I'm from a very big family – my mother is one of seven and my dad is one of five, for starters – so I had plenty of relatives who used to babysit for me when I was small. Overnight visits at my aunts' houses were part of the fun, and I always looked forward to them.

Things changed a bit when diabetes came into the picture. Sleepovers weren't as easy to manage, because now we had to juggle insulin injections, blood sugar tests, and being on the lookout for high and low blood sugars – especially back in that first year when everything diabetes-related was so new to all of us. I was still a little kid, and now all this medical stuff, too?

When I was first diagnosed, I didn't do my own insulin injections. At the outset, my parents did my injections for me, but after a few months, my extended family started to learn. I think about it now, having baby-sat for my nieces and nephews and little cousins, and I can't even picture that learning curve. I'm so grateful that my family came together to learn to deal with diabetes, instead of leaving my mom and dad as the only ones capable of care.

One of my earliest memories with diabetes is of me waiting on my aunt's couch while my mother tried to explain to my aunt how to administer my insulin injection.

"You need to uncap the syringe, check for any air bubbles one last time, and then pinch up where you're going to stick the needle. Once the needle is in, you press down the plunger and pull the needle out. No problem!"

My young aunt was nervous. "I pinch the skin and then put the needle in? How fast do I put the needle in?"

"Pretty quickly," my mom responded. "Don't think about it. Just jab it in there, as gently as you can."

"Okay, so pinch, jab, plunge, remove. Got it."

"Great, so are you ready to give it a try?"

The entire time they're debating this, I'm face-down on the couch with my pants halfway pulled down, waiting for the insulin injection to be given into the top of my seven-year-old butt cheek.

My aunt came towards me, brandishing the syringe like a hot fireplace poker. She uncapped it nervously, pinched up the top of my hip, and said, "Ready, Kerri?"

"Yessh I amph." I said into the couch cushion.

"Okay, here we go!"

She expertly stuck the syringe needle into my skin, and I barely felt the pinch. And then she pulled the needle back, letting out an, "Oooh! I did it!"

My mother sighed.

"You didn't push the plunger down."

"What?"

"The plunger. To dispense the insulin? You didn't push it down. You just stuck her with a needle and then pulled it out again." I could hear my mother trying not to laugh.

"Oh shit!" my aunt exclaimed.

I giggled at the curse word, despite the fact that they were about to advance on me again with that syringe.

"You shed de esh word."

Stings

It was fifth grade. Mrs. Henry was our language arts teacher. It was the first year we had lockers and they were situated outside of her classroom. It felt cool, having a locker. We cut out pictures from Tiger Beat magazine and hung them on the inside of the door. Melissa, my locker partner, and I cut out pictures of tropical fish and made our locker an 'aquarium.' She even made a fake aquarium filter out of a used water bottle and some aluminum foil. Peak fifth grade art.

Melissa, Hannah, and I were walking back from the cafeteria after lunch and we stopped by our lockers to put our lunch bags away. Hannah grabbed her reading book from the top shelf of her locker. Melissa didn't need anything because she already had her book. I reached into the bottom of our locker to retrieve my reading book and saw a folded-up piece of paper stuck in the locker vent.

"To Kerri Only."

"A note! Kerri got a note! Oooohh…" Fifth grade immaturity gave way to giggles and blushing as the three of us crowded around the note to read.

"Dear Kerri, the Dirty Diabetic. No one likes you. We've made a whole club about how we don't like you. It's called the 'We Hate Diabetics' club."

A picture of a needle encased in an accusatory red circle was scribbled beside my name.

Melissa and Hannah stood there, not saying anything. Until I started to cry.

"That's not right. That's mean! We're taking this to Mrs. Henry. She'll find out who did this." They took the note from my hands. Then they took my hands in theirs and led me into the classroom.

The note was handed to Mrs. Henry and she read it while Melissa rummaged in her pockets for a tissue for me.

"This is unacceptable." She shook her head and her soft blond hair swished from side to side. "This is simply unacceptable."

Through the miraculous methods that only 5th grade language arts teachers possess, Mrs. Henry found out who has left that note in my locker. The "We Hate Diabetics Club" consisted of a red-headed girl I knew from lunch, whose eyes were red-rimmed as she shuffled towards me at the urging of Mrs. Henry's hands.

Red Head stopped in front of me and stared at her feet.

"I'm sorry, Kerri," she mumbled, looking to Mrs. Henry to release her from apologetic duty.

"It's okay," I said back, looking for her to release me.

Red Head remains the only person in my life who has ever tried to make me feel bad for being diabetic. She made me cry and, when I think about the moment I opened that note, I'm still surprised. I wish I could forgive her for her childish words, but I still can't. She and I continued through middle school and high school together, attending the same parties and dances and mixing with the same group of friends, but I always held her at arm's length. And when I saw her at the beach last summer, after a decade of distance, I didn't walk over to say hello.

Even if I want to pretend it doesn't, it still stings.

Clink, Clack, Clink, Clack

The sounds of my childhood with diabetes, the bottle of NPH as my mother rolled it against her wedding rings. Every morning, she would wake up at 5 am to get ready for work, stopping by my bedroom to test my blood sugar. Even though I was still asleep, the sound of her approaching slippers made my finger automatically stick out from underneath the mountain of blankets. She would then roll the NPH to mix it up in preparation for my morning injection.

Clink ... clack ... clink ... clack.

The glass bottle rolling against her rings in the early hours of my school days. The stale, hollow beep of my old Accu-Chek meter after it had counted for 120 seconds in efforts to offer up a result. The scratchy sounds of the cellophane wrapper on my Nabs crackers, or the rustle of the straw piercing into my Capri Sun. The hot fizzing of the urinalysis tablets as they cackled from their glass test tubes on the bathroom counter.

These are the sounds of my childhood with diabetes.

Now, as I have become an adult, there are new sounds that define my diabetes life. The boop *beep* **boop** of my insulin pump as it administers a lunch bolus. The *whirring* of the pump as it primes itself. The sharp *thwarp* of the lancing device as I prick my fingertip. The chalky scrape of glucose tabs rustling against one another in the jar. The gentle clicking of the beads on my medic alert bracelet.

These sounds have replaced the diabetes ones from my childhood. I wonder what sounds twenty years from now will bring.

Even though I now use Humalog insulin that doesn't need to be mixed, I'll roll the bottle against my rings and to remember.

Diaries of a Diabetic Girl

I last cracked the binding on my old journals years ago, when I was cleaning out the apartment I was living in at the time. I happened upon them again last night, while searching for something in the attic. (I never found what I was looking for up there, but I did come down with a bunch of stuff I *wasn't* looking for. Going into the attic is like going to Target.)

These journals span the better part of ten years, starting from when I was about eight years old and going into my junior year of college. They're old and tattered; it's fun to flip through them and see what was top-of-mind for a ten-year-old. In the earlier journals, diabetes is rarely discussed. There are mentions of attending Clara Barton Camp, but nothing really specific about diabetes or insulin injections or any of the tasks I knew I was tending to at the time. (I was busy being "just a kid" and not "a kid with diabetes," which is the kind of childhood I was happy to have.)

But one entry, from back in 1999 when I was in college, talks exclusively about diabetes, and the period of burnout I was experiencing.

> "I have been diabetic for 13 years (this September) and I don't know if I've taken the best care of myself. I have eaten a lot of the wrong things. I don't exercise enough. Even though I still test, I am reluctant to test and last week, I saw a 50 and a 350 in the same day. Not okay. I hate taking my insulin shot. I'm really scared of lows, especially after the one when I couldn't find the honey jar fast enough. My A1C runs at levels that makes my doctor raise an eyebrow sometimes because she knows I've been thinking about having a baby someday. I went to the Joslin Clinic last Thursday and they said I need to start thinking now about having babies much later.

Which is hard to think about, since I don't even have a father for these not-yet-made babies. Am I screwing up my chances of having a baby by having trouble controlling my diabetes? It's a weird place to be in, worrying about stuff that won't happen for a really long time, but that's how diabetes is – makes you worry about all the crap in the future that other people might not think about until it's actually happening. Must be interesting, not banging your head against a crystal ball all the fucking time."

I wish I could send that girl a note, the 20-year old me who wrote with painstakingly neat handwriting (shocking, compared to the scratchy EKG graph my pen produces now), and tell her that just a decade or so later, she'd be sitting at her kitchen table and drinking coffee, having just sent her three-year-old daughter to preschool for the morning.

That even after crossing the line into "complicated," it's still okay. The payoff seems irritating at times – "Work hard and the reward is ... to keep having to work hard?" – but the alternative is unacceptable. Life with diabetes often means trying, and continuing try, even when you don't want to.

I'd also suggest that she stop cursing so much back in the day, because surely, she'd kick that habit as an adult.

Surely.

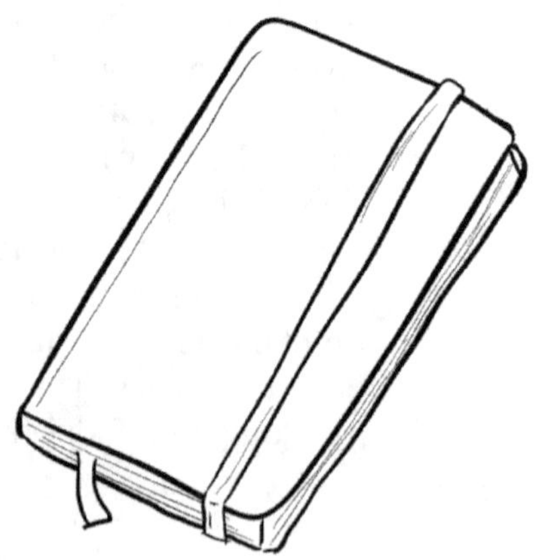

What Happened at Lunch ("Sorry, Mom.")

After my elementary school diagnosis with diabetes, my school lunches were ruled by the American Diabetes Association exchange program. The version I used looked like a meal card plan without any wiggle room, listing the food requirements for each meal. Lunch, for example, included two starches, one protein, one vegetable, one fruit, one milk, and one fat exchange.

Looking at this list now, I see things like carb counts and insulin-to-carbohydrate ratios, making meals seem like options and not force-feeding to chase the spike of NPH insulin. But back then, meals were carefully structured to meet the peaks of my insulin, and my mother took great care in planning my lunches so that my blood sugar wouldn't tank during the school day.

I'd leave the house each morning with a brown paper bag that contained some combination of my exchange combinations, like a turkey and cheese sandwich (two starches, the milk, and meat, with the lunch meat weighed on the food scale at home) with some mayonnaise spread on the bread (the fat), a bag of carrot sticks (vegetable), and a pear (the fruit).

And my mom was probably feeling pretty secure about the whole thing, knowing that she dosed me with my morning insulin shot (a mix of Regular and NPH) that would work to cover my breakfast and then the lunch. What happened at lunch, theoretically, is that I'd eat what she packed and birds would sing and squirrels would jig in jubilant step with one another and my blood sugar would be 104 mg/dL when I came home in the afternoon.

What really happened at lunch was that, like any other kid at school lunch, it wasn't about eating your lunch. It was about trading food.

Which meant that my mom's carefully packed lunch, coordinated with my insulin dose and my food exchange to best take a bite out of type 1 diabetes, sometimes ended up being traded for Ring Dings and a piece of pizza. I felt bad about it, at the time (and still now), but I distinctly remember trading a plastic sandwich bag containing white rice cakes smeared with peanut butter for someone's Yodel (oh, Yodels). It was a normal lunchtime trade for the other kids, but for me, it was like the black market for snacks, gaining me access to the forbidden fruits and Yodels that my parents avoided having in our home.

In retrospect, I was following "the exchange system" too literally.

Most days, I ate what my mother packed for me, but on those days when I caved to the middle school bartering system, I went right off the rails. And then I'd marvel, alongside my mother, at the high blood sugar I'd be hosting when I came home from school. "I have no idea why I'm so high."

As a kid growing up with type 1 diabetes, I had the chance to make more than my fair share of less-than-optimal management decisions. But it's the guilt that made its way into my adulthood more than the impact of those off-days.

I'm thankful that the insulin options, both in actual insulin and delivery, have progressed to make meals times less stressful. At least then I would have had the wherewithal to bolus for that Yodel.

The Curse of the Camp Coleslaw

"Your meal card says you need to eat one vegetable and one fat. This coleslaw is your vegetable and your fat." My camp counselor sighed, having been through this routine with me before. "You need to eat it. You can't leave the table until you've eaten it."

"But I haaaaaaate coleslaw!!!!" I wailed, eight years old and wearing my tie-dyed Clara Barton Camp t-shirt.

When I was small, I went to summer camp. Only my summer camp was specifically for girls who had type 1 diabetes. It was just like everyone else's summer camp, only at mine, we did drugs before breakfast. (Insulin, ya'll.) But we also had strict meal plans, suggested by the American Diabetes Association, that needed to be followed to the letter, as our insulin doses (NPH and Regular) and meal plans were planned to be in sync with one another. One step out of turn and blood sugars would bounce all over creation.

As an eight-year-old, I didn't have the most daring culinary palette. A yummy meal, to me, was grilled cheese and sugar-free lemonade, followed closely by strawberries and Cool Whip. When presented with things like hard-boiled eggs and avocado, I'd hide behind the dining room curtains. (My feet stuck out at the bottom, so I was never hidden for long. If you had told me then that, as an adult, I'd love hard-boiled eggs and avocado – together! – I would have laughed myself right out the window.)

Food wasn't a means to a blood sugar end, or even something to explore and enjoy. Food was something I needed to eat, and fast, before I could go back outside and play. It was very Machiavellian.

But the rules at camp were unbendable. My parents trusted the camp staff to keep me and my complicated disease safe for two weeks in the summer, and the camp staff took that responsibility very seriously. Without insulin that acted faster than Regular (no Humalog back in 1988 and carb counting wasn't a best practice yet), I was forced to stick with the meal plan.

"I do NOT like coleslaw! It's slimy! And gross!!" I crossed my arms over my chest, indignant and frustrated that most of my fellow campers were already up and exiting for Flag (the ceremony where we lowered the flag at night). Most campers ... except for me. And my friend Liz, who also refused to eat that coleslaw.

"The faster you can eat it, the faster we can go out with everyone else and have fun. Can you just take one bite?" (Looking back, I don't envy the position of the counselors, having to cajole little kids into eating nightmare-textured foods.)

"Fine." I shoveled three bites into my mouth at once, and washed it down with huge gulps of water. "It tastes horrible!"

"Keep going ..."

And on we went, laboriously, until the side of coleslaw was eaten and I was released from the dining hall. Force-feeding (aka "clean your plate!") was a common occurrence back in the early days of my diabetes, since insulin and food were so acutely dependent upon one another. I am thankful for the treatment progress I've seen over the last few decades, from insulin delivery methods to actual insulin.

But I still won't touch the 'slaw.

Chopping Broccoli

I'm the middle child of three, the only one in my family with type 1 diabetes. Diabetes influenced food choices for the whole family, but we weren't without sweet treats, especially since my brother and sister weren't under the thumb of NPH and Regular insulin.

So sometimes my mom got crafty with her food storage stylings in efforts to keep super sweet foods out of my diet but within reach of my siblings.

Like when she'd buy boxes of frozen broccoli,

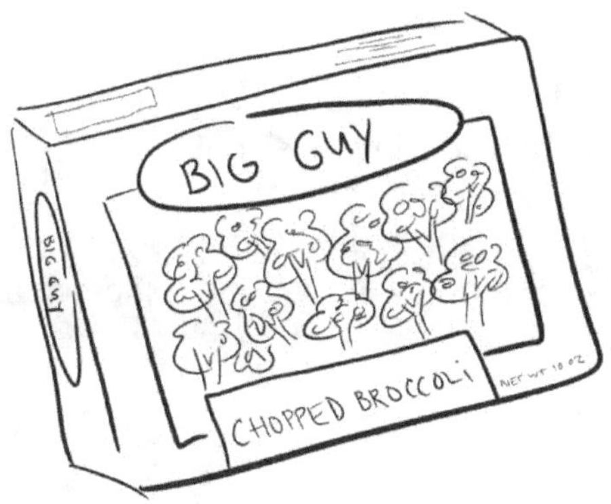

and take out the broccoli,

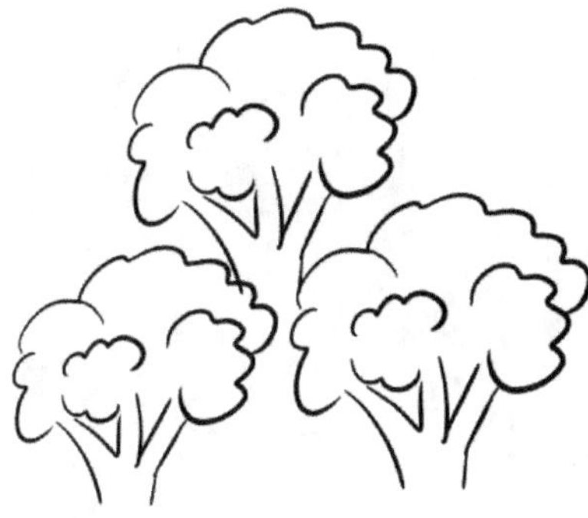

and replace it with ice cream sandwiches.

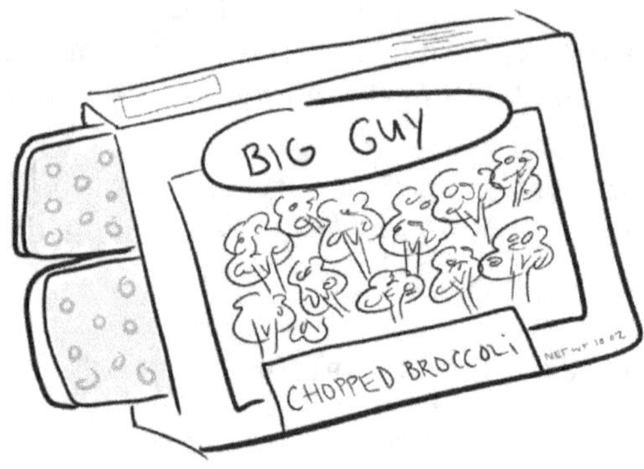

My mom did what she could to keep things as smooth as possible at home, taking care of all three of her kids back in 1986.

Every time I think about this bit of protective repackaging, I appreciate the work my mother did to keep it as normal as possible.

Between Dinner and a Movie

Saturday nights when we were very small were the best.

We made blanket forts and used every damn cushion in the couch. Setting pillows on the floor, we'd jump from polyester-filled island to island, pretending that the carpet was infested with alligators and only by balancing on the pillows would we be safe.

The babysitter always promised to make healthy dinner, but usually we ate popcorn and chicken fingers, and drank diet soda by the bottle, filling the glasses to the very brim and frantically slurping the carbonated foam away before it could spill over.

My favorite babysitters were the ones who played with us, not just sat there and talked with their friends on the phone. Carolyn was my favorite one of all and I named my favorite Cabbage Patch doll after her. She was athletic and smart and the characters she invented when we played were so clever. She was the perfect example of what a 'hero' really was, to my seven-year-old self.

My parents had a standing Saturday date night, and they would go out to dinner either alone or with some friends, then maybe to a movie. Usually, they left when it was still light out, while we were still outside playing in the yard or just coming in to have a snack. My brother and sister and I played and fought and made messes and told stories and generally destroyed the house, like kids do.

Only now, when my memory is jogged, do I remember the headlights pulling back in the driveway, between when dinner ended and the movie began. Dad would wait in the car while Mom ran in quickly to check my blood sugar and give me my bedtime insulin injection. Then she'd say goodnight to all of us and run back out to the car to continue date night.

Only now do I remember those moments and wish I'd named my Cabbage Patch doll after my mother, instead.

More Than Candy and Costumes

Dressing up was not an issue. I wore my silly costumes proudly and they were always homemade. I was a fairy godmother one year. I was a fortune teller for about three years running. Another year I was Bo Peep, complete with sheep.

Then one year, I was diabetic.

When the central focus of the holiday is eating candy, what's a kid with diabetes to do?

I can't admit that I remember it being a big deal, but my mother will recount that first Halloween, when she leaned in to give me a kiss and she smelled chocolate on my breath. "I thought it would kill you," she admitted. That panic, that first taste of fear was something my parents felt so I wouldn't have to. I was just a little six-year-old kid. I was more concerned about whether or not my costume skirts were getting tattered on the edges from running through the streets on Halloween night.

In the first few years after my diagnosis, the candy was monitored and handled by my mother. I had a few pieces, a little bit was stashed away as "reaction treaters," and my brother and sister bartered with me for the rest. My older brother, little sister, and I would sit on the floor after trick-or-treating and pour our pillowcase collections of candy out onto the floor, separating the candy into genre piles – one for chocolate, one for hard candies and gum, and a potluck of the non-candy items like pencils and stickers.

It's no coincidence that I ended up with all the pencils and stickers as my brother and sister grinned at me with chocolate-stained mouths.

I used to sneak pieces of candy, though.

I remember finding the reaction treatment stash and cramming five or six mini-Snickers bars into my mouth. The chocolate taste was sickeningly sweet and tasted like delicious deception. I didn't get caught but the feeling of guilt I experienced is something I can still feel deep in my stomach if I think about that moment too much.

I had diabetes, but you couldn't tell by looking at me. In my group of friends, you couldn't pick me out of that crowd. Which is probably why the police officer made use of his police cruiser intercom to harness my attention.

I was about nine years old, trick-or-treating with my friends in one of their neighborhoods. There were seven or eight of us and we were all costumed and toting pillowcases to carry our bounty.

The headlights came up behind us first, then the swirling red and blue police lights. The intercom squealed on.

"Kerri Morrone?"

We stopped dead in our tracks. No one turned around. My friend Christie whispered loudly to me, "Did they just say your name?"

"Kerri Morrone? We're looking for Kerri. Is she with you guys?"

My blood ran cold. What could I have possibly done? Did they know I talked during the D.A.R.E. presentation and they were mad about it? Did they find out I had pinched my sister on the arm for telling on me? Oh my God, did they know I sneaked candy every Halloween?

Like a convict on the run finally giving in, I turned around slowly and raised my hand over my head.

"I'm Kerri."

The intercom squealed to life again. "Please come over to the car."

I shuffled my shoes, now filled with lead, toward the police cruiser. My friends stood back, clutching their pillowcases and staring.

The window of the police car lowered and revealed the smiling face of Officer Mark, the young D.A.R.E. officer who visited my middle school every fall.

"Hi, Kerri. Sorry to scare you." The grin on his face was warm and friendly. "You know, my wife is diabetic. She likes this special sugar-free candy. I thought, since you were diabetic too, that you might like some." He reached to the seat beside him and handed me a white box with a black and orange ribbon tied around it.

Are people aware of the very moment they affect your life forever? The moment that they make you feel less alone?

"Thanks, Officer Mark. Really, thank you. This is awesome. I thought I was in trouble, though!"

His grin became even wider. "Yeah, well you're not. But make sure you and your friends stay out of it!" He leaned out the window and gestured toward my friends. "Be careful, girls! Have a good night!"

"Bye, Officer Mark!!" they all called in unison.

The next year, I dressed up as a fortune teller ... again. I was also still a diabetic.

I was okay with being both.

Your Mama is So Awesome

Your mama is so awesome that she dragged measuring cups and a tiny scale to restaurants so she could accurately carb count your food.

Your mama is so awesome that she hand-fed graham crackers to you while you had a logic-defying low on the kitchen floor.

Your mama is so awesome she woke up in the middle of the night to check your blood sugar, to keep you safe and to keep diabetes from waking YOU up.

Your mama is so awesome she took time off from work for all the field trips, school events, and overnights so that you would be carefully monitored without missing out on the fun.

Your mama is so awesome she drove home between dinner and the movie so that she could check your blood sugar and give you insulin.

Your mama is so awesome that she said "We need to check our blood sugar" because despite the lancet not pricking her skin, she still felt her version of every number.

Your mama is so awesome she gave you your insulin shot even though you were hiding behind the dining room curtains, even though you cried, even though it was hard.

Your mama is so awesome she sought out and sent you to a diabetes camp so you could find your community and feel a different-but-necessary sense of home.

Your mama is so awesome that she only kicked a hole in ONE blue bin that ONE time.

Your mama is so awesome also because she continues to call your CGM a "GPS."

Your mama is so awesome that when you were pregnant and stayed over at her house, she came into your room in the middle of the night to try and make sense of the Dexcom receiver and the data it was providing.

Your mama is so awesome that she was mad when you told her that the blog posts can be set to auto-publish. "That's how I knew you were okay every day! I didn't know you could write them ahead of time!"

Your mama is so awesome she calls you while your husband is traveling to "see if you watched the TV show" but she just wants you to answer the phone and confirm your continued existence.

Your mama is so awesome that she came up to the hospital the first time you had a c-section in part because she wanted to meet her granddaughter but also because her baby was having an operation and she wanted to be there.

Your mama is so awesome that she watched that granddaughter so you could go have another c-section to bring her grandson into the world.

Your mama is so awesome that she hears your meter BEEP or the Dexcom wail and doesn't freak out, but casually stares at you without making it seem like she's staring until you grab some juice, God damn it.

Your mama is so awesome that when you think about growing up with diabetes, you aren't saddled with overwhelming memories about feeling different, or unsupported, or defined by this disease. Instead, you remember the life that diabetes is part of. And you've carried that mindset into adulthood. You can make some sense of this disease because she supported, and continues to support, the whole of you.

Your mama is so awesome.

What Helped Me as a Kid with Diabetes.

I was diagnosed with diabetes in second grade, so I've had this disease along for essentially all of the available rides in my almost 40 years. From 1986 onward, I've experienced everything from field trips to fights with my parents about boyfriends to learning to drive to college to pregnancy and parenting children of my own. My life, for all intents and purposes, has always included diabetes.

And for the most part, I think I've had my wits about me in terms of this disease.

When I travel to speak at conferences and advocacy events, parents of kids with diabetes regularly ask me a version of the same question: "What did your parents do RIGHT when raising you with diabetes?"

It's a tough question. My bias of love towards my parents is hard to shake, and I also know they were/are not perfect. (Same goes for me – no perfection here.) They're good parents. From the diabetes perspective, a few specific things were very helpful:

Diabetes counted when driving. When I was preparing to get my license, it was 1995 and glucose meters were able to provide a memory bank of checked glucose numbers. A condition my parents set for earning my license was that I had to check EVERY time I got behind the wheel, and straying from that plan meant I couldn't drive. And I wanted to drive SO VERY MUCH that I was willing to do anything to earn that independence.

As a result, I checked my blood sugar constantly. And also offered to go pick up milk anytime we needed it, even twice a day, if necessary. This habit has served me well into my adult life, only now I check my CGM before I drive.

I had independence when seeing my clinician. When I was a teenager, my mother started splitting the appointments with my endocrinologist with me. We'd go in as a team for half of the appointment and then she'd step out for part of it. This allowed me to stretch my own wings as a patient, raising any concerns I had without worrying what my parents would think. This was especially helpful when I was considering becoming sexually active, because it allowed me to have honest conversations about risks, prevention, and sexual health with my doctor, helping me make informed decisions as a young adult.

I was encouraged to seek help. When my parents divorced when I was 20, my overall health took a swift nosedive and my diabetes was no exception. During this emotionally loaded time, I was encouraged by my parents to seek help from a very skilled psychologist who specialized in type 1 diabetes, and her intervention kept me from making some less-than-optimal decisions. This interaction proved to me that my emotional and mental health needed as much support as my physical health, a realization that served me well when I experienced postpartum anxiety after the birth of my son.

It was not an excuse. Diabetes was not an excuse in my household. It wasn't a reason not to clean my room or avoid my homework. Diabetes wasn't a reason for talking back to my parents or being late for curfew. It wasn't this get out of jail free card for being an asshole to people. I was sometimes punished for diabetes-related things, like lying about my blood sugars or not checking when I said I would.

And while I hated being held to a standard that no one else in my family had to manage, I realize that my parents made diabetes something I was taught to take responsibility for, and not something to crutch out on. Now, I appreciate that diabetes was included by my parents on my list of "chores" because that put diabetes management into a silo of non-negotiable, accept-it-and-keep-at-it things.

And I wasn't alone. Early on, my family sent me to diabetes camp, allowing me to connect with other kids who had diabetes and who understood what it was like to feel like "the odd man out." Finding my peers, especially at an early age, showed me that diabetes wasn't rare and wouldn't hold me back on the whole, and for the moments when I felt overwhelmed and isolated, I had my diabetes camp friends as an emotional boost. This goal of peer connection clearly carried on for decades, as I've been writing a diabetes blog for almost 14 years now.

I mess things up on the regular. But diabetes, for better or for worse, has been so tightly woven into everything I do that it doesn't feel like an intrusion. An inconvenience? Yep. Something I out-and-out loathe from time to time? Hell yes. Something I appreciate the perspective I've gained from? Fine, I'll admit a yes to that one, too.

There's always been an ebb and flow to the measure of grace I've approached this disease with, and perfection hasn't ever, and WON'T ever, be achieved. Nope. And my parents and I fought regularly and aggressively about all kinds of crap, including diabetes. But through hard work and a refusal to let diabetes define me, my parents helped me make this disease a capital T "Thing" but not an all caps "THING." And if I had to do it, I'd approach parenting a child with diabetes similarly.

Thanks, mom and dad, for helping me become an adult who can mostly handle her stuff. I promise to try and clean my room more regularly now.

Twenty-Five Years with Diabetes: What I've Learned.

What I've learned in the last twenty-five years with type 1
diabetes:

- Some of what "they" said is wrong. It just is.
- There are times when "they" make a good point, and it's
  up to us as patients to figure out what information we
  react to.
- The needles don't hurt as much now as they did then.
  Lancets have become smaller and sharper, syringes can
  make the same claim. Insulin pump sites, once they're in,
  usually go without being noticed. Same goes for Dexcom
  sensors. (But "pain free" is a misnomer and so subjective
  that medical device advertisers had best just steer clear of
  that word entirely. All needles pinch at least a little bit.)
- Progress isn't always shown in tangible technological
  examples. Sometimes progress is being able to look at a
  blood sugar number without feeling judged by it. Or to
  look in the mirror without wishing you were different.
- There is life after diagnosis.
- Diabetes is sometimes funny. It has to be. If I didn't find
  ways to laugh at this shit, I would cry more. And crying
  leads to dehydration, which is a precursor for ketones,
  which aren't fun. So ... that brings us back to "diabetes is
  sometimes funny."
- Diabetes sometimes **isn't** funny. Sometimes this is the
  most serious disease in the world. It's a strange balance,
  acknowledging both aspects of this chronic disease.
- "Comfort food," to me, is a jar of glucose tabs on the
  bedside table when a blood sugar of 43 mg/dL wakes me
  up in the middle of the night.
- It's okay to cry about diabetes stuff. It's okay to celebrate
  the victories, too. This is life, and it's okay to feel all parts
  of it.
- Food wasn't for fun or nourishment for many, many
  years. Most of my childhood was spent viewing food as
  medicine; the means to an NPH peak's end.

- I am grateful that I've learned to eat because I'm hungry. Or because it tastes good. Not just because I "have to."
- Some days I feel like a steel magnolia. Other days I feel like a wilted tulip. Diabetes and flower similes aren't my strong suits.
- Diabetes scares me. To my very core, sometimes. I hate admitting that. I hate fearing something that I have inside of me every day, something I can't shake in any way, shape, or form. It's unnerving, never truly letting down my guard.
- Diabetes scares me most when I think about how it may affect my child. Which gives me a different perspective on what it was like for my parents. Which makes me want to call my mom and dad and say "thank you."
- Diabetes also inspires me. Same; to the core. It makes me work harder, fight longer, love harder, appreciate more.
- Family isn't limited to those in your gene pool.
- Testing my blood sugar is the best way for me to keep tabs on my diabetes. I wish I could say that wearing a pump was the answer, or using a CGM, but those devices are tools. Effective tools, but still just tools. I achieve the best outcomes when I test my blood sugar and actually respond to those numbers, both mentally and physically.
- Everything in moderation. Including platitudes. Turn the other cheek to platitudes.
- It took me a really long time to realize that perfection wasn't an achievable goal. Diabetes isn't a perfect science, and you can't hit the bullseye all the time. Maybe not even half of the time. The goal is to always aim for it, and to keep trying.
- It took me just as long to realize that diabetes-related health complications aren't my fault. Diabetes complications are the fault of diabetes, not of me. My job is to keep trying. (See above.)
- The word "diabetic" hasn't ever bothered me. (Maybe because I'm lazy and I don't want to say "person with diabetes"?)

- The word "complications" doesn't just apply to retinopathy, renal issues, and neuropathy. Diabetes is complicated in so many ways outside of the reach of a test result.
- Emotional health is just as important - maybe more so, to me - than physical health. Diabetes is a disease that requires your head to be "in the game" in order for your health to be optimal. Emotional health needs to be nurtured just as acutely as your blood sugars need to be tested.
- I've learned that I am not alone.
- Let me repeat that: I am not alone. And if I'm not alone, then neither are you. We are in this together. And we can do this.
- Success with diabetes, for me, isn't a perfect A1C. Or a crisply organized logbook. It's not a week's worth of no-hitters. Success with diabetes, for me, is feeling happy. Despite, because ... whatever. Just feeling happy.
- And I feel like I'm succeeding.

Thirty-One Years with Diabetes

When my diabetes marked its 25th birthday, I wrote a bulleted of stuff I've learned since diagnosis. (See previous essay.) Another handful of years later, most of that list still holds up, with a few tweaks:

Sometimes I can't believe this is still a Thing, like capital T Thing. That diabetes is still a thing that requires attention, work, and patience. I used to believe in the "five more years until a cure" rhetoric, but that promise has been folded and refolded six times over by now. I believe that the research maybe prevents diabetes in my children, but I'm not sure it will cure it for me. And that weirds me out. "Forever" was always tempered by that, "Yeah, but in five more years …"

There's a strange sense of acceptance that's come in the last seven years, accepting that diabetes might not really be cured for me. I find myself looking at research and technology that's rocketing towards alleviating the burden of diabetes on people living with it and feeling encouraged by that progress. And it's not just the big, known companies who are making a difference. It's the smaller, renegade start-up ones. And the community groups. And the people with diabetes who are empowered and inspired to make a difference.

I'm regularly impressed by families who live with diabetes. They know how to take These Things seriously without taking those things **too** seriously. They speak in a special language of numbers and ratios and tubing lengths and lab work percentages. They are tireless, even when they're tired.

They inspire the absolute hell out of me.

Life is still filled with a whole bunch of colors and I'm not done coloring yet … even if it's occasionally outside the lines. Despite diabetes. And because of diabetes.

But admittedly, I still do not like this disease.

Yep. I can't pretend to be above that, to have embraced it and found happiness in it. Nope. I do not like diabetes. Any grace that's borne of it doesn't change the chokehold it's had on my life at times. I wish that wasn't true, but it is true.

However. I have to acknowledge what I've gained as a result of this disease.

Not just perspective, although that's a powerful grab. Troubles whittle themselves down a little bit when put through the mental diabetes woodchipper. That perspective has been to my benefit as I went through my teen years (other girls were angry and upset that their jeans were a size 8 instead of a size 2 – I was fine with a size 8 so long as my morning BG was between 80 – 110 mg/dL) and also as I managed pregnancies (stretch marks, morning sickness, yeah, but that I made that healthy baby).

I've also made friendships – ones as chronic and lifelong as diabetes – where these like-pancreased connections are part of my inner circle for life. These connections were forged through similar circumstances but will remain intact despite distance, time, and even a cure.

The reality of diabetes sets in more and more, especially as the same realities of regular life hit their stride. I can't pretend that it's all easy and effortless. This shit might look easy, but some days it's hard.

Diabetes scares me more now that I'm older. I read about heart attacks and other crisis events and used to think, "Damn. They were so young." And now I read, thinking, "Damn. I'm in that age range where I'm old enough for it to happen and young enough for people to think, 'Damn, they were so young.'"

This freaks me out. I worry about the big things more these days than I did before. I try not to, but I still do. Sometimes bedtime is when my brain hits the spin cycle and I have trouble falling asleep, picturing what-if scenarios.

Aging and diabetes are also flagged concerns. Are my knees making that weird cricking sound when I run up the stairs because I'm older? Or because of diabetes? Or is it a combo deal? And when you answer, can you speak up because I'm seriously having trouble hearing you.

Even after 31 years, diabetes still has days where it behaves. And days when it doesn't.

I can say exactly the same for myself.

Since I wrote my list at 25 years of diabetes, I've had another little baby bird and my life now is tied to two young people. I have two kids to stay healthy for, two kids to annoy well into their old age. The motivating force towards good health that my children provide cannot be properly appreciated. They are my little world.

My hope lives in a different house now. As I mentioned, I'm not expecting diabetes to be cured, but I'm anticipating that I may be able to ignore it altogether in the future; that data and technology will come together in a way that doesn't make me produce insulin but also doesn't produce worry and anxiety in the same way. Stick on the device and it will diabetes (a verb) for you.

Yes, please. Hurry, please.

I hope for my kids. I hope for their kids. I hope that my mom will know with certainty that diabetes will never make my life any less **mine**. I hope that my husband knows I'm working to be healthy for decades to come. I hope the community rallies and sticks together with one another, rising up against our common enemy while educating, supporting, and loving one another. Enormous thanks to all of you for being part of a network of hearts and hopes that make this walk with diabetes easier, and less lonely.

After 31 years, I look at this body, all riddled with shouldn'ts and can'ts, and see that it should, and it can. And it will.

A Letter to a Younger Me

Dear Littler Me,

I wish you'd known you weren't alone. That even though you didn't have a bunch of friends with diabetes (YET) when you were growing up, you still had lots of friends. And a family that loved you. And people who didn't understand exactly what it meant to be "low" or "high," but they wanted to, and they tried.

I wish you had known that there were other kids just like you. It wasn't until you spent your summers at Clara Barton Camp that you realized just how normal diabetes was for some families. That some kids woke up every morning, just like you did, and shot up. Or that some kids were hounded by their parents to "just let me check your pee for ketones, okay?"

I wish you had known that doctors bend the truth a bit. That when they said, "This won't hurt a bit," it was going to hurt anyway. That when they promised not to draw blood from your arm unless your parents were there, they lied and instead stole into your hospital room at 1 am and woke you up with their midnight vampirism. I wish you had known that when they said, "Kids may not be in your future," you didn't have to believe them.

I wish you had known about the impact of sorbitol and other sugar-substitutes on your little kid tummy. Dude, that stuff will wreck you up right proper. And for days.

I wish you hadn't written those notes on the backs of school quizzes and then stuck them into your Bible for safe-keeping. The ones that included long diatribes about how some girls in your class didn't understand. Or about how you were 385 mg/dl and you had eaten the cupcakes you claimed to have ignored, and you wish you felt brave enough to confess to your mom. I wish I didn't find those notes 18 years after the fact. I wish I hadn't remembered how isolated and guilty and scared I felt at those times.

I wish you had known that, despite the excuses you wanted to make, that every day matters. I'm glad you know it now, but I need you to remember it more. Every day matters, Kerri. Yesterday may not have been the best diabetes day, but today can be better. Stress and work and vacations and traveling and motherhood will always be there. You need to learn how to dance between those raindrops and still give your health the attention it deserves.

I wish you had known that pumping insulin was going to be an easier transition than you thought. I know you were scared about having an "external symptom" of diabetes, and worried about the implication of "robot parts" on your dating life, but it wasn't an issue at all. (Your husband hasn't ever known you without the pump - who would have thought?!)

I wish you had known, in that moment of diagnosis, that it was going to be okay. There are ups and downs with everything, and diabetes is part of that ebb and flow, but there is life to be lived - a good life - even with diabetes. You have some extra issues to deal with as a result of this disease, but you will be okay. Remember that, especially when you feel overwhelmed now, as an adult. Don't lose hope, even in that cure that's been promised to you five times over now. And don't, for crying out loud, let any kind of pity party overtake who you are.

I wish you had known that you CAN eat that, and you CAN do that, and you CAN work there, and you CAN love him, and you CAN be loved back, and you CAN be happy. So go DO and BE, kid. Enjoy every minute, because it goes by in a blink.

Love,
Future You

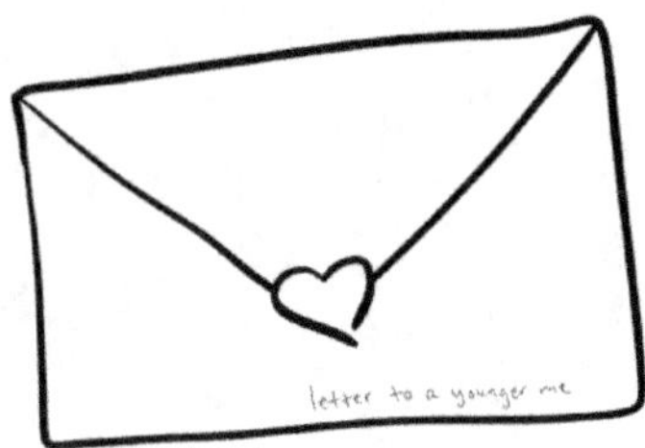

Diabetes in
the Wild

Diabetes in the Wild

I see people with diabetes everywhere.

I spy their insulin pump tubing sticking out from underneath the edge of their shirt. I see the continuous glucose monitor sensor on their arm. I can hear the telltale beep of their devices from across a crowded subway car. (And if I see a grown human being drinking a juice box with any air of desperation, you can bet I'm making some hypoglycemic assumptions.)

Seeing someone else with diabetes gives rise to this instant connection. You KNOW things about one another, things that even the people who are closest to you aren't aware of. Like what it feels like to be low, when the thoughts just won't come and you're at the bottom of that mental well. Common experiences make strangers less strange.

In the last two decades of diabetes-related conferences, traveling, and community engagement, I've had the chance to meet so many other people with diabetes. These moments are so important in normalizing diabetes for me; we're all out there, living our weird lives together. And even in the unrelated-to-diabetes day-to-day moments, I'm finding diabetes in the wild.

The connect is cathartic. It's a moment of magic. We build bridges of humanity and understanding with little more than a knowing glance and an empathetic smile.

These essays are about seeing diabetes in the wild, making connections, and feeling less alone.

The Droid You're Looking For

I grabbed the Dexcom receiver from my purse and gave the button a quick click while I was standing in line for coffee, checking the graph and noticing the single up arrow, pointing my blood sugar up from 146 mg/dL.

A moment of mental math took place: I was rising, but I had some insulin on board, and how many carbs was I about to consume? After a quick calculation of the insulin I had on board already, I reached underneath my shirt and grabbed the insulin pump off my hip. Buttons pressed, bolus delivered, but whoops – ended up a bit tangled when I went to clip the pump back to my hip and I ended up flashing the infusion set on my hip by accident.

The guy behind me in line was there with his son, who had started first grade a few weeks ago. (How do I know this? Because when they got into line behind me, the little boy smiled at me and said, "Hi! I started first grade last week!") It wasn't until I had successfully untangled my pump and returned the Dexcom back to my purse that I realized the little boy was staring at me with wide, blue eyes.

"I learned a word last week in first grade," he said to his father, tugging on his sleeve insistently.

"What did you learn?" the father replied absently, as he foraged for his wallet.

"'Droid.' It means you have robot parts. Like Luke Skywalker's arm after his dad cuts it off! And the yellow C3PO guy! And that lady!" He pointed at me.

"What?" The father was paying rapt attention now.

"She has droid parts. I saw them." He smiled, sticking his tongue through the hole where his front tooth should have been.

"Ethan, that's not nice. Apologize to the lady – she's not a droid."
The father looked at me and said, "I'm so sorry! He's watched a
lot of Star Wars. Like, a lot," with hands on his son's shoulder.

This is where I should have given a nice, concise speech to this
little boy and his father about diabetes and the hardware
involved. This is where I should have said, "Oh, I'm not a robot.
I'm wearing an insulin pump and a continuous glucose monitor
and I wear these devices because my body doesn't produce a
hormone called insulin." There are many things I should have
done at that moment.

But instead, I grabbed my coffee from the counter. I smiled at
Ethan. And I leaned down to whisper, "I'm not the droid you're
looking for."

His whole little kid face lit up and his words came out in one,
single, excited breath. "*Oh-my-gosh-Dad-she-knows!*"

PWD in the Wild

We were sitting at the coffee shop having a really nice Melbourne cappuccino (they make the best cappuccinos I've ever had in my whole life, with the steamed milk almost like a marshmallow topping on each coffee - amazing), talking about the Australian diabetes social media summit. The weather was sunny and crisp, with plenty of other patrons enjoying their caffeine jolt at the outside cafe tables.

"I guess when I was diagnosed, it didn't matter much to me that I didn't know anyone else who had diabetes. I didn't really know what diabetes was. But as I grew older, I wanted to find that community, and that's where the Internet has helped tremendously," I said to Renza, talking about the impact of the diabetes community on my emotional well-being.

"And here we are now," said Renza, laughing as she stirred her coffee.

We chatted on about the Summit the day prior, and what we thought of it. And then our conversation tumbled into our personal experiences with diabetes and pregnancy. Thinking back on this conversation, we probably said the word "diabetes" at least a dozen times in a ten minute conversation.

Which is probably why the young woman was staring at us from her table, just a few feet away. She was holding her coffee cup near her mouth, but hadn't had a sip yet. She was fixated on our conversation. Her young daughter was drinking a frothy mug of hot chocolate, swinging her feet as the wind caught and tousled her bangs.

"Excuse me," she said, almost to herself.

My seat was facing her table, so I leaned in and said, "Hello!"

"I couldn't help but overhear - you both have diabetes?"

Renza shifted in her seat. "Yes, yes we do. I'm sorry - were we being too loud?"

The woman laughed nervously, the cup still close to her mouth but merely an accessory at this point. "No, not at all. I was happy to hear ... I mean, my daughter was just diagnosed with type 1 diabetes a few weeks ago. We've never met anyone else who has diabetes." She made a sweeping gesture with her hand. "And here you both are!"

"Real life people with diabetes, in the wild," I smiled.

Renza leaned back and extended her hand, introducing herself and explaining to the woman that she had type 1 diabetes and also worked down the street at Diabetes Australia Vic. "You can come visit us any time you'd like - and I'm at this coffee shop all the time." She handed the woman her card.

Thank goodness for the poise and professionalism of Renza. I couldn't help myself; I waved animatedly at the girl and her mother and this stream of information passed my lips: "I'm Kerri and I live in the United States and I've had type 1 diabetes for twenty-six years and I have a husband and he and I have a daughter who is two and a half."

I wanted them to know I was okay, and that even though my life has included type 1 diabetes for several decades, I was still okay; it was a consolidated diabetes life story in one messy sentence, delivered with a caffeinated edge.

"How are you doing? How are you both doing?" I asked.

The woman looked at her daughter, who was staring at us. "We're good. We're doing good. We come to this coffee shop often because they are the only ones who really listen to how I want her hot chocolate prepared. Her daycare is right around the corner, so it's a nice place to stop. They do listen ..." her voice trailed off.

"We do know."

We talked for a few minutes, and the woman gathered up her belongings. "It was so nice meeting both of you. Really. Thank you." Her daughter stared at us with her big, brown eyes, the same as her mother.

"Our pleasure. I hope to hear from you. Please do reach out," said Renza warmly.

The woman took her daughter's hand and crossed the street toward the daycare center, her delicious Melbourne coffee still untouched on the table but every single sip of her daughter's special-made hot chocolate devoured.

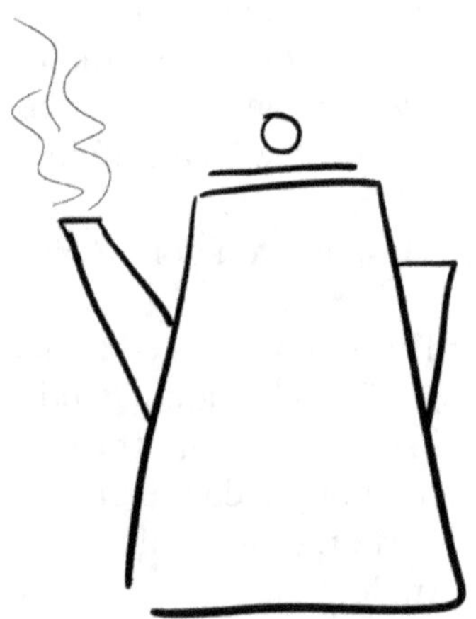

Insulin Pump on the Beach

"Oh, it's like what Cindy has! That's what Cindy has!"

The lady was about twenty feet away from me, stage-whispering to her husband.

"Is that the pump? The insulin pump thing?" her husband asked, gesturing toward me.

I lifted the beach blanket by its corners so it would spread out nice and flat. "It is an insulin pump," I said to them, waving, unaware until that moment how obvious my insulin pump was, clipped to the bottom of my bathing suit, the tubing tucked in kind of haphazardly. "It's nice to meet you!"

The woman came over, her hands fluttering and her mouth talking and smiling all at once. She was so excited ...

"... to see a real insulin pump! My daughter went on one a few years ago, but I've never seen anyone else with one. And at the beach!! She's going to love hearing this. Your pump looks different from hers - is it?"

(I loved that she automatically assumed I knew what kind of pump her daughter was on, as if there was a community of people with diabetes who are in constant contact with one another and comparing notes ... wait a second ...)

"Mine is an Animas pump. Is hers Animas or Medtronic? Does it have tubing?"

"Yes, it has the wires. Hers is the Medtronic one. She really likes it. How long have you had diabetes?"

"Twenty-five years. How about your daughter?"

"About twenty years. She's 31. She's trying to lose weight and be in better control. I don't know half of what she does, but I know she's always trying to do better." The corners of her mouth tugged into a brave smile. "She doesn't know I worry but I worry all the time."

"My mom does, too." My mother and Birdy were a few yards away, building a sand castle. "She worries. But she knows I'll be okay."

"Is that little one your daughter?"

"Yes. She's two."

The woman smiled. "My daughter would like to have a baby. That's part of why she went on a pump. You know."

Birdy came running toward me, her ponytail bouncing and covered in sand. "Ocean, Mama!!" The bucket of sand in her hand spilled as she lifted her arms excitedly. "Sand! I has sand!"

I gave the woman a big grin as my daughter tornado toddled up the beach, her arms outstretched.

"I do know."

The Friendly Skies

"Hi there. Are you the guy who is responsible for this section of the plane?"

He was holding a tray of drinks and paused to contemplate my question. "I suppose I am. I am responsible! Now I feel powerful!" He flexed, as much as he could in the limited corridor.

"Awesome. I don't mean to trouble you, but I am traveling alone and wanted to let the closest flight attendant know that I have type 1 diabetes. Not a big deal, but just something to have on the radar if I were to have an issue of some kind."

I don't mind traveling alone – sometimes, when it comes to the chaos of TSA and luggage and all the rest of it, I prefer alone – but when I am literally flying solo, I feel a little vulnerable. I always wear my medical alert bracelet when I'm away from home, but sometimes that doesn't feel like enough. And for this particular trip, where I'd be in the same plane seat for upwards of seven hours on an overnight flight, I wanted to make sure someone had diabetes in the back of their mind, just in case.

"Not a problem at all. Type 1 or type 2?"

(What?)

"Type 1, diagnosed when I was in elementary school. Do you have diabetes in your family?"

"My brother was diagnosed when he was eleven. Lots of shots, lots of all of that growing up. But he's doing just fine now. Two young kids, one more on the way."

"Aw, good for him. So you know it better than most, right?"

"I'd hope so, after sharing a house with him and our parents for so long. Do you mind if I ask what your symptoms are, for your reactions?"

"Honestly, you'll know something's up if I start crying without cause, or if I go pale and shaky, and have a hard time communicating."

"Does the light go out of your eyes, too?"

It's funny how only those who know, who have seen hypoglycemia in their personal lives, understand what that means. How low blood sugars make the light go out of your eyes, makes them empty for that brief moment.

"That's it. That's it exactly."

"Well," he said, resuming his semi-flex and throwing out a reassuring grin, "as the one in charge of this part of the plane, I can assure you that you are in good hands. No trouble at all – we'll keep an extra eye on you."

"Thank you so much. I really appreciate it."

We continued on to our final destination without diabetes incident, and I was again reminded of how small the diabetes community is, and how understanding it can be, down to the smallest detail.

McDave from the Plane

"Were you saving these seats for us?"

I travel regularly for work, and because I'm usually on the road without my family, various discussions with strangers fills in the quiet spots. Since my days as a breakfast waitress in college, I've always enjoyed those snippets of single-serving conversations, like they talk about in Fight Club. Airplane travel can offer insight at 30,000 feet.

"Yes. I've been waiting for you guys for hours," I replied, standing up so that the couple could join me in row 9.

This was my introduction to Dave and his lovely wife. Throughout the course of the flight from Orlando back up to Providence yesterday, I spent some quality time talking with these two and over-sharing to a potentially dangerous degree.

We talked about flying, and how none of us cared for it. We talked about the Patriots and how my mother and his wife are intensely passionate fans. We talked about how his daughter has been an extra in several films and TV shows. And we talked a lot about food.

After a discussion about what I do for work and what brought me into the diabetes space (see also: diagnosed 28 years ago, felt alone, founded a blog, found some friends), Dave admitted that his own diet could use a shift in priorities.

"We could eat better," he said.

"We could eat a LOT better," his wife added, from the window seat, furrowing her brow.

"Everyone could eat better, but our fast-food society doesn't exactly make it easy. You have to go above and beyond to make sure you aren't eating junk. Junk is mainstream! Think about how screwed up our perception of 'breakfast' is; we dump sugary syrup onto pastry-esque pancakes and call it a healthy meal. That's not a meal … it's dessert!"

They nodded, and I realized I was on a mile-high soapbox. "I'm so sorry. Food stuff makes me ranty sometimes. Like when I think about the kinds of foods marketed towards my daughter. Chicken nuggets and French fries and sugary cereal. Stuff is gross."

"So she's never had a Happy Meal from McDonald's?" asked Dave, half mocking me, half actually asking.

"She's had McDonald's food two or three times in her life, but that's it. And no, she's never had a Happy Meal."

He laughed. "You're missing the chance to make her happy! But not the food – I get that you don't want to give her the food. I used to make my own Happy Meals for my daughters. I'd take a toy that they hadn't played with in ages and pack it in with their lunch. Instant Happy Meal!"

"That's a good idea. I like that."

"Yeah. Now you can write about it in your blog website, right? I want to be in there. People would want to read more about me."

His comments made me laugh. "Sure. I'll write about you. But the blog post has to have some kind of resolution, right? Where we both promise to make changes and then we hold one another accountable? Or is that taking it too far?" I asked him.

Dave thought for a minute. "I can do that. Listen, my wife and I will make a change. We promise to eat something green with every meal. A vegetable, like spinach or broccoli or squash. Except that squash isn't green, so we'll have to be flexible with the color requirement. But a vegetable with every meal." He made a fist and jabbed it towards the air with conviction. "A vegetable with every meal!"

"And I promise to make my kid a happy meal, like the one you described."

He handed me his business card and I promised to send him a link to the blog post once it was live. The plane landed and we all went our separate ways, resolute in our decisions to make positive changes.

This morning, as I packed Birdy's lunch for preschool, I put one of her small, forgotten toys in the lunch bag, alongside her healthy food options (and a cartoon drawing of the cat drinking a mug of steaming coffee). I wondered what kind of vegetable Dave managed to work into his breakfast that morning.

What's the point of going through life without ever making eye contact, or making a connection? Single-serving or not, I'm better for having sat next to Dave.

We Made Contact

The Starbucks on the ground floor of the hotel was a busy one, with conference attendees, hotel guests, and Philadelphians streaming in from the city street, all clamoring for their cup of coffee.

My friends and I stood in line to order, then shuffled over to the "holding area," where we waited for our over-priced coffee to be doled out. Some people sat in the window seat, some stood and tapped their feet impatiently. I leaned against the high bar behind me, watching the baristas whirl and spin around each other like socks in the dryer.

That day, I was wearing pants and had my pump clipped to my pocket. Because I was in a hurry to get back up to the conference, I had run to the bathroom first, and then trotted over to Starbucks. My pump tubing, though usually tucked away, was flopping outside of my pocket and dangling towards my knee.

And this lady kept looking at it. She was sitting on the window seat, so my hip was right in her line of vision. And she just kept looking.

I caught her eye. "Hi." And smiled.

"Hi." It was like she couldn't help herself - her eyes darted back down to my tubing. She smiled apologetically.

"It's an insulin pump?" I said, like it was a question I was asking her.

"A what?"

"An insulin pump. For diabetes?"

"Oh! I didn't mean to stare. I just thought it was your cell phone, but then I saw that tube hanging out. For diabetes?"

"Yes. Instead of taking injections of insulin, I use the pump to administer it throughout the day." We both looked at the tubing. "I like it."

"My daughters - they're your age - keep telling me to get an iPhone. 'Get an iPhone, Mom! You have to!' But I don't want one. I don't want that much technology. I just want my phone to make phone calls, you know?" She gestured towards my pump. "But if I had diabetes, that's the kind of technology I'd want. I'd want that."

Her coffee came up on the bar, and mine quickly followed.

She paused a second. "Most people in the city don't make eye contact."

"That's kind of sad. But look at us! We've made both eye contact and pump contact!"

"Eye contact and pump contact. This has been a unique morning!" She grabbed a few napkins for herself and, out of habit, I think, handed me one for my coffee. "Have a good day, sweetie, and take care of yourself."

We made contact.

Overnight Flight Discussion

After an unexpected overnight in the airport in Baltimore, the passengers of flight #627 were finally queued up for their flight home. I was sitting in the seats closest to the windows by gate A5, drinking some water and bleary-eyed with exhaustion.

The guy next to me was wearing sunglasses and a hat, worked over by the evening's chaos.

"Did you get your new boarding pass yet?" he asked me, nodding to the line of people at the customer service desk, waiting to be reissued boarding passes for the new flight.

"I did. I went out and back through security, because I figured it would be quicker." I gestured towards the staggeringly long line. "I think I did the right thing."

"Security isn't fun, though. All that unpacking and repacking and the shoes and the bitching and moaning ... everyone's always unhappy, and no one can get through without a hassle. I once had a piece of gum in my pocket, and the scanner picked it up. Something about the aluminum in the wrapper. Such a pain."

"I hear you. I wear a medical device, and it can cause a party at the security lines at times."

He took a knowing sip of his coffee as he looked at my hip. "Insulin pump?"

"Yeah, how did you know?"

"You're young, you look healthy, but you mentioned a medical device. I figured it was an insulin pump." He proudly tapped his shoulder. "Diabetic for seventeen years. Only I do shots. My doctor keeps talking to me about the pump, but I'm not there yet. I work outside, and in construction, and I think it would be in the way."

"I did shots for seventeen years before switching to a pump. I don't know; I like mine. It took some time adjusting to physically wearing something, but for me, things are just easier when I have it handy. I can sleep in, or skip meals ... gives me a lot of flexibility."

"So you like it?"

"As much as you can like robot parts, yeah."

He smiled. "Doesn't hold you back or anything?"

"I don't think so. I've worn it camping. And hiking. And in swim-up bars on vacation. And on my wedding day. And while I was pregnant with my daughter." I laughed. "And now I've worn it for an impromptu no-sleep-sleepover in an airport. Adventures!"

"I have some bad lows. Man, you just don't KNOW how bad a low feels until it's right on top of you. I've had some at work that have made things really tough, until I can get my hands on some candy. I try to explain it to my coworkers but they just don't know." His voice broke on the word *know*.

I smiled as gently as I could. "Well, I know, if it helps. That's part of why I went on the pump, because I was having some really insane lows in the early morning hours. It was really ugly, and dangerous."

"Maybe I'll check it out for real at my next appointment. I see my doc next month. I'll tell her that a random girl at the airport convinced me to get an insulin pump."

"Or you could blame sleep deprivation."

We talked about the Dexcom (he wore a blinded one for a week, on the recommendation of his endocrinologist; I said that I rarely, rarely take mine off), about watching our kids for signs type 1 (compared notes on testing their blood sugar at random), and the effects of travel on diabetes (sustained chaos for both of us).

The flight attendants called us to line up to board the flight, and as we were gathering our belongings together, he touched my shoulder.

"It was nice talking to you. I don't get a chance to talk with other people who have this thing, too, but it's nice to do that. I liked doing that."

"Same here, man. Enjoy the rest of your trip!"

I never caught him name. Didn't need to.

So Much Bigger

I took two packets of sugar substitute from the basket near the coffee maker and flicked my fingers against them to loosen up the granules, then ripped open the paper packets and poured them into my coffee cup.

"What kind of insulin pump is that? My grandson has an insulin pump."

His voice was warm and kind, and he stirred his own coffee absently, looking curiously at the pump in my pocket.

"An Animas Ping." I smiled at him. "How long has your grandson had diabetes?"

"A little over a year. I like your pump. It looks small. What kind is it, again?"

"Animas. What does your son have?"

"Medtronic." He looked at my pump again. "It just looks so much bigger than that one."

"I think most of the tubed pumps are generally the same size, give or take. Mine is about the same size as your grandson's. How is he doing with it?"

The grandfather smiled. "He does great. He's a good kid. He was on the pump soon after being diagnosed. His grandmother and I are here at this conference to learn all we can and report back, since his parents couldn't come because they're home with him."

He paused. "Are you sure your pump isn't smaller? It looks a lot smaller."

"I'm almost positive."

We both sipped our coffees.

"How old is your grandson, sir?"

The smile on his face flew like a bird from his mouth to his eyes, though it was a bit sadder when it landed there.

"He's two. Two and a half."

My insulin pump was the size of a whisper, sitting on the hip of a grown woman, compared to being clipped to the pajamas of a two-and-a-half-year-old boy.

My eyes filled with tears that I ignored as I sipped my coffee as a distraction. "The pumps are the same size. It's the size of the person wearing it that varies, I think."

"That must be it," he said. "But still. Everything just looks so big on him."

Airport Connections

The plane from Cincinnati to Washington, DC was a teeny one, leaving little room for carry-on luggage and even less for calm.

After ferreting out my medication bag from my suitcase, I checked it at the gate and ended up second-to-last to board the plane.

"Smells like … something, doesn't it?" The gentleman behind me asked casually. I wasn't sure if he was addressing me, but I answered anyway.

"It does. Like a ham sandwich. Or Bad Thanksgiving," I replied, noticing that the plane had a "stale cold cuts" smell to it.

We boarded the small plane and took our seats at the back of it. Turns out the scent-sitive man who boarded behind me was also my seatmate.

We chatted briefly for a few moments about what we did for work – he worked for a surgical medical device company, I told him I was a writer – and then the discussion turned specifically to medical devices.

"I'm familiar, to a certain extent, with some medical devices. I wear a few for diabetes management," I said. "Going through TSA is always interesting."

He looked at me for a minute. "Diabetes? Type 1?"

"Yes. Since I was seven years old."

"My daughter is nine. She also has type 1."

And over the course of our flight to Washington, DC on the plane that smelled like spoiled lunch, this kind man and I compared notes on life with type 1 diabetes from our different perspectives.

It wasn't a life-changing moment or a pivotal interaction, but served to confirm once again, how diabetes becomes a common thread that brings strangers together.

Even on a stinky plane.

Close, But(t) Not Close Enough

"My mom? She has brown hair and a red shirt," said my daughter's playgroup friend, climbing up the jungle gym.

"My mom is over there. She has a pump in her butt," my daughter pointed towards me and waved, causing me to quickly answer the look of surprise on the other parents' faces with a brief, panicked explanation of the insulin pump connected to the top of my left hip.

America Runs on Insulin

It's been well-documented that my coffee addiction is ... substantial. Briefly on hiatus during my pregnancy, I was reunited with my beloved beverage after the baby was born, and now I'm back in the habit.

Since I work from our home office and I'm also the primary caregiver for Birdy, sleep is a hot commodity. Actually, I don't get to sleep much, so the coffee is very much my friend these days.

Work hard, play hard, drink much of the coffee.

The other day, I was out with the baby, running a few errands. I had to visit the post office, the grocery store, CVS ... and Dunkin Donuts. I try to make my order sound fresh and new (versus something I say almost without thinking), and I leaned out the window to order into the drive through speaker. (Instead of into the garbage can, which is something I've done more times than I'd care to admit.)

"Hi!" Total joy. "Can I please have a medium iced coffee with cream and two Splenda?"

"Sure thing. Please drive up."

I drive up. But when I get to the window, there's a little bit of confusion.

"Okay, so one coffee with milk and sugar, two doughnuts, and a bagel with cream cheese?" The boy attending the window had a bag of deliciousness in his hand. My stomach said "YES! YES. THOSE BELONG TO ME."

I mentally punched myself in the stomach and said, "Oh, I only had a medium iced coffee. That was it."

"No problem." The kid put down the order that wasn't mine and returned with a single iced coffee. "Okay, that's two dollars and thirty-six cents."

"Awesome." I handed the money out the window. "Would you mind double-checking to see if that's with Splenda, and not sugar? I'm diabetic, and I don't want to end up with the wrong order."

He paused. "Type 1?"

Whooo boy.

"Yes, type 1."

"Yours is definitely Splenda. I'm positive." He handed me my change. "My mom has type 1. For like, ever. How are you doing?"

This kid wasn't any more than 18 years old. But the concern on his face was wise beyond his years.

"Good. I'm doing really well. I've had it since I was a kid."

"My mom, too. She's doing good. And she has me. And my sister. Is that your baby?" He waved at Birdy in the backseat, waving her chubby arms around and babbling.

"Yes. She's almost a year old. It's refreshing to see that our kids grow up to be nice kids."

He smiled. "And that our moms weren't always old moms. Have a good day. And I can't wait to tell my mom I met another one like her."

People with diabetes are everywhere. And so are the people who love them.

"Bag got run over."

I'm not a light packer, but I am an efficient packer, in that I can fit a week's worth of clothes, diabetes supplies, and travel needs (laptop, sundries, phone, etc.) into a carry-on bag. I hate checking luggage. But for this last trip, the total time away was ten days (and included several days at a conference with "real shoes' and 'real dresses' instead of casual clothes), so I had to buckle and check a bag.

But I still kept all my essentials (read: meds and technology) in the roller carry-on bag, to protect my diabetes supplies from the cold of the cargo hold and the possibility of being lost. See? Responsible-ish.

Which is why it sort of sucked when, as Chris and I were putting in the code to enter the building of the apartment we had rented in Paris, a box truck rolled by at the same time as a guy on a bicycle. And in the chaos, my carry-on bag pitched into the sidewalk and was run over by the truck.

"Oh," I said, kind of casually, watching as the first set of the truck wheels crunched over the handle of my bag, crushing it.

"Oh shit," I said, less casually as the bag pivoted a little bit and the truck wheels further obliterated the handle, coming so, so close to smushing the contents of my bag.

"Bag got run over," I said to Chris, half in disbelief and half channeling a neanderthal.

We both stared at it, and realized at the same time that my pump supplies, bottles of insulin (Humalog and Levemir), test strips, back-up meter, and all my insulin pens were in that bag. Along with my laptop. I immediately, and thankfully, thought about the global diabetes community and how, even in a foreign country, I could hopefully connect with other people living with diabetes and borrow enough insulin and test strips to hold me until I was able to claim a stash of my own.

Nothing to do but drag the broken soldier into the apartment and assess the damage. Miraculously, the truck only destroyed the elongated handle of the bag and dented the very top of it, leaving everything inside still assembled. A week's worth of diabetes supplies were safe.

And it dawned on me that even the best laid plans can still become a big, fat mess. Because even though I had packed enough supplies to brace me for a broken bottle of insulin, or gaffed up pump, or lost meter, I hadn't split those supplies into more than one bag, leaving everything I needed to sustain my life in one, vulnerable spot.

"Good thing it didn't smash the bag," I said, pulling out my laptop and inspecting it for damage. "My laptop would have been destroyed. Oh, and all my insulin. Both needed for my nerdy survival, right?"

Lesson learned: Next frigging time, I'm splitting my supplies. And steering clear of traffic.

Pumped for the Pizza Man

The oven broke.

It took me a while to notice, because it was upwards of 90 degrees inside of my house (no central air ... we will not be making this mistake with our next house), but once I realized the stove was kaput, it was about 6.30 pm and very much time for Birdzone's dinner. While I'd like to say that I walked out to our garden and picked enough fresh green beans, tomatoes, and lettuce for a healthy salad, then followed up with chicken on the grill, with a dessert of fresh blackberries and cream, I can't.

Because I never ended up planting the garden I wanted to (too much time on the road) and we don't have a grill (still haven't bought one) and the frigging birds keep snaking our blackberries so, to this day, I haven't had a single blackberry from the huge bush outside due to the aforementioned shitty birds.

So we ordered a pizza. Judge all you want.

Birdy and I were playing in her air-conditioned room when the doorbell rang, signaling the arrival of the pizza man.

"The pizza man is here!" Birdy opened her door and let in the dragon-breath heat from the kitchen, scurrying towards our front door with her yellow Batman Princess tutu flapping at her waist. I handed her a few dollars so that she could tip the delivery person.

I opened the door and the guy handed us our pizza and drinks.

"Here you go, miss. It's hot, isn't it!" It wasn't a statement, but a declaration, as the heat was undeniable.

"Yeah. Our stove broke, so there was even less of a chance of me cooking."

He smiled as Birdy said, "Hi!" from behind my legs and darted out to hand him the money.

"Thank you … um, Batman," he said, slightly confused but offering her a friendly smile.

"You're welcome!" and she took off. I thanked him, and shut the door. A few seconds later, the doorbell rang again. (The pizza man always rings twice?)

"Hi again. Sorry, but I forgot to have you sign the debit card slip." He handed me a slip of paper, and as I signed it, he asked, "Do you have diabetes?"

"Excuse me?"

"Diabetes. Do you have diabetes? I noticed the sticker on your car said 'insulin' or something on it, and I wondered if you were diabetic."

I laughed, surprised. "Yes, I do have diabetes. Type 1, diagnosed as a kid. Do you?"

"Yeah. Diagnosed as a kid, too." He reached into the pocket of his cargo shorts and pulled out a Minimed insulin pump. "I've been pumping for about six years."

I lifted the corner of my shirt and flashed him my silver Animas Ping. "Almost ten years for me. Small world! And that sticker on my car is for Insulindependence. It's a diabetes organization focusing on sports and exercise."

"Cool – I'll check it out," he said, winding his pump tubing around his fingers as he shoved the pump back into his pocket.

"Cool." I paused, and the words tumbled out like I was confessing. "I don't normally eat pizza, you know."

The pizza man grinned. "It's like the most complicated bolus ever. No matter what, I never get it totally right." He started to walk back towards his car, waving at Birdy. "Have a good night! Stay cool!"

Birdy appeared from behind the door. "Mawm, he had a pump, too! He has diabeedles!"

"He does!"

The diabetes world is a small, small one. Never before had I been so pumped to see the pizza man.

(Yes. We went all that way for a horrible pun.)

Hawkey Playah

I clicked the button on my Dexcom receiver and saw a "212 mg/dl" with two arrows pointed straight on up. This was the third effortless high in as many hours, and I was convinced my pump site had crapped out.

"I am going to run to the bathroom. I need to switch out my site," I said to Chris, moving my napkin from my lap to the table. "Do you mind sitting here ..."

"At this giant hibachi table all by myself? Sure," he grinned, gesturing towards all the empty seats.

"I know. I hope this table fills up while I'm gone. Otherwise, this is going to be awkward, just us and the hibachi chef guy." I patted his shoulder as I stood up from the table, the small, gray inset tucked into my hand.

I am not a fan of doing site changes outside of the comfort of my home. When I'm at home, I prefer to put the new infusion set, insulin cartridge, the bottle of Humalog, and any other necessary accoutrements on the bathroom counter. I like looking in the mirror to see where the site is going to end up, because I have specific preferences as to where it lines up with the waistband of my pants or the sleeves of my shirts.

Picky little parsnip that I am, I like putting my new sites on in a measured manner.

When it became clear that my pump site has conked out on me and needed to be changed immediately, my first thought was, "thank goodness I carry a purse big enough to throw a spare set into," and then "Oh shoot – now I have to do this in the public bathroom?"

I went into the ladies' room and was greeted by very dark lighting, two large stalls, and no bathroom counter. (The sink appeared to be suspended in midair. I think it was deliberately trying to mess with me.) I casually went to the stall and disconnected the infusion set from my arm.

The cannula was piped with blood, so I knew it was definitely uncooperative. I set the pump to start rewinding, and the BUZZZZZZ of the pump motor echoed in the empty bathroom.

"Man, that never sounds so loud at home," I said to myself.

I finished disconnecting and rewinding/priming the pump, and I stepped into the hand-washing area of the bathroom so I could use the mirror to line up my new site. I pulled up the back of my shirt enough to see my hip, and then placed the inset against my skin.

And then bathroom door opened and a friendly-looking woman came in, just in time to see me pressing the buttons on the inset, pushing the infusion set needle into the skin on the top of my hip.

"Oh, I'm sorry!" she said. "I didn't mean to interrupt ... what ... whatever you're doing."

"No worries." I felt a little embarrassed – nothing like being caught with your shirt all gathered and a needle in your side. "I am a diabetic and I have to fix my insulin pump. I needed to use the mirror ... it's totally a medical thing." The words flapped out of my mouth like spastic birds.

She walked over to get a better look at what I was doing. "Insulin pump? My brother is a diabetic. Has been for almost twenty years. He's forty and just got married. I'm having dinner with him right now!" She smiled and gestured towards my pump. "I wish he'd go on that thing. He's been doing shots for like ... evah. He has thought about a pump but he hasn't done it yet."

"Whatever keeps you healthy is best, right?" The new infusion set shot in with a quiet *shunk*, and I tucked the pump back into the pocket of my jeans after taking a correction bolus.

"True. He's done this for a long time. He and his wife are talking about having kids. Do you have kids? Can you have kids?"

"I have a nine-month-old. She's happy and healthy. And so am I."

The woman put her hand to her heart. "Oh doll, that's wonderful. I hope my brother can have kids. He'd be a good dad. But if he goes on a pump like you've got there, he'll have to be careful with it. Gettin' it knocked around, you know? He's a wicked hawkey playah."

"Hockey is awesome. Give your brother my best, okay?"

Back out in the dining room, a quick look at the Dexcom showed me that the correction bolus was working, and that the new site was on track. And from across the crowded room, I saw the woman sitting at a table with her group, the wicked hawkey playah at her side.

The Mothership

"Mom, that lady has special powers and is an alien. I know because I saw her alien transmitter in her pocket and it has wires and it talks directly to her body using that tube. I saw it. She can't hide from me because I saw it and it looked that's how she communicates with the mothership but she's safe and she didn't seem scared, right?"

It's at that point that I felt the need to explain to the eight-year-old boy's mother that it was an insulin pump.

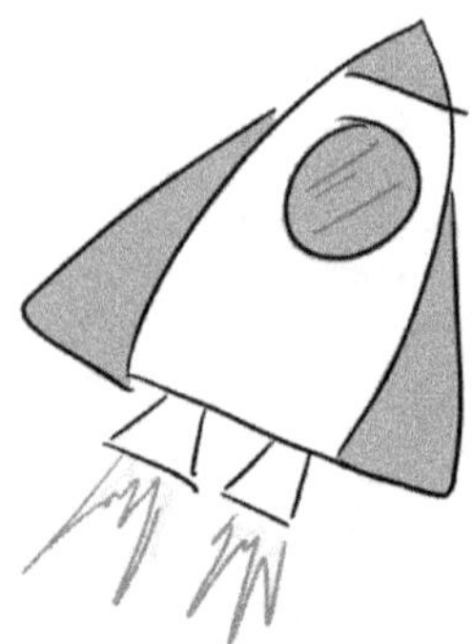

These Boots Were Made for Talking

I was coming home from Washington, DC and my flight to Rhode Island was delayed. The wait in the cramped US Airways terminal was long and oddly warm for October, giving people a certain irritated twitch. I was still dressed from my meeting, with a dress, tights and boots and not enough real estate in the dress itself to hide my insulin pump so eff the bullshit, I clipped my pump to the top of my boots. It felt comfortable and somewhat subtle.

The other people on my flight and I kept close to the gate, watching the delay extend and hearing sighs from fellow travelers. There was a thick tension to the air, one that even the smell from the Dunkin' Donuts kiosk couldn't cut through.

Suddenly, a fight broke out between these two random ladies, one of whom was heavily pregnant. There was excitement and a scuffle and lots of "Oh no you did NOT" and the response of "But I DID." Security showed up around the same time as our plane, which added to the chaos.

"This was unexpected," the man next to me said, shaking his head.

"Almost makes the plane delay tolerable," I agreed.

He looked at me and then his eyes traveled to the top of my boot.

"Is that an insulin pump?" he asked, with a look on his face that indicated he was familiar.

As I said, "Yes," I realized that I meet people touched by diabetes everywhere. In coffee shops, at Disney World, on planes, going through TSA, and now, watching a pregnant lady and another lady try to punch one another in the face while waiting for a delayed plane. People with diabetes are everywhere, and I am lucky to find a lot of them.

... that, and it probably helps catalyze conversation, keeping my medical device clipped to my shoe.

"My daughter has type 1 diabetes," he said. "She was diagnosed when she was nine. She's 18 now and at college. Volleyball player," he added proudly.

"No kidding? I've had it for 29 years, diagnosed when I was seven."

"Yeah? Wow, 29 years." He looked impressed, as if I had mentioned an ability to build functional spaceships out of pasta noodles instead of an inability to produce my own insulin. "And you're okay?"

I shrugged, thinking about the difficult last few months. But I was okay. I'd be more okay in time.

"I'm not picking fights with pregnant people at the airport, so I'd say I'm pretty okay."

He looked at me with those hourglass eyes that parents of children with diabetes often have, visibly fast-forwarding his own daughter's life another two decades, wondering what her life would be like when she had lived with diabetes for almost thirty years.

"That's a plus," he said.

And all at once, I wanted to give him a run-down of my life, telling him everything that I had still done and would still do, despite or because of diabetes. I wanted to show him pictures of my daughter. I wanted tell him about how Chris takes care of me without smothering me. I wanted to tell him how my mom and I are immeasurably close through diabetes. I wanted to tell him it would be okay and his kid would be okay.

And then I wanted him to tell me I would be okay, and that the people I love who have diabetes would also be okay.

The gate attendants called for people to start boarding our flight. We shook hands and did the "Nice to meet you; good luck with everything" send off.

But there was a moment that hung between us, one of understanding and connection that only people who really understand this life can share.

Diabetes Shorthand

Last night, my oldest kid and I went out for a mommy-and-daughter dinner date. Our waitress was a student at the local university, and very nice.

She took our order ("Wow, your kid chooses broccoli over French fries! I'm impressed!") and then turned to go back to the waitstaff station.

"MOM," Birdy stage whispered at me. "She has a Dexcom on her arm."

I looked over and, sure enough, there was a G6 Dexcom sensor visible just beneath the sleeve of the waitress's short-sleeved shirt.

"Oh yeah! I see it!"

"Are you going to tell her you wear one when she comes back?"

"Sure, I can do that."

The waitress came back over and brought our drinks. "I noticed your Dexcom; I wear one, too."

Her face brightened. "Hey, that's awesome! I like it wearing it on my arm. But you know, sometimes I have trouble keeping the sensors stuck."

We spoke in diabetes shorthand for less than a minute, comparing favorite adhesive overlay tapes and body real estate options. She pantomimed carefully putting on a shirt to show how sometimes her sensor gets stuck on the sleeve hem. I pantomimed pulling down a pair of pants by exaggeratedly stretching out the waist to show how to avoid pulling off the sensor from my thigh. She told me about the random guy at a bar who showed off his insulin pump after seeing her Dexcom sensor. We laughed at the absurdity of the whole robot-life thing.

My daughter watched us, two strangers fluent in the same foreign language.

We ordered our meal. It came, we ate it, and we paid the bill. I left an excessively large tip because college students with diabetes are paying for more than just books.

We're everywhere. These chance encounters, these shared experiences where two people with diabetes take a minute to speak that experiential diabetes shorthand and share a moment of connection ... they are what make this greater diabetes community remarkable.

Unexpected Advocacy

The last thing I wanted to do was take off my cover-up.

Chris and Birdy (and our friends and their daughter) were at a water park in New Hampshire where kids can run and play in safe-for-littles sprinklers, pools, and water slides, and as the adults, we were tasked with guarding the perimeter. Pacing back and forth, the four of us kept watch on our kids, ready to jump in at any moment to help them climb a slide, pick them up if they fell, or slather on more sunscreen.

I didn't care who saw my body. Not really, anyway. I've run miles and given birth (not simultaneously), so I know there are strengths and weaknesses to my frame, but it wasn't the shape and curve of my body that made me want to stay covered up at the water park.

I didn't want people staring at the diabetes devices stuck to my body.

"Oh for crying out loud. No one is looking at you."

Of course, they aren't. Or at least they don't mean to. But when someone walks by wearing a bathing suit with a few curious looking devices hanging off it, it's hard not to notice at least a little bit. My standard beachwear is a bathing suit with my pump clipped to the hip, the tubing snaked out to wherever the infusion set happens to be inserted, and my Dexcom sensor taking up more skin real estate elsewhere. These items aren't enormous, and people don't snicker, but they do look twice because cyborgs are still somewhat rare.

Most of the time I don't think twice about who might look, but on this particular day, I felt self-conscious. Why? Who knows? Who cares. I was in my own head that day, and feeling like hiding.

But motherhood dictated that my feelings take a backseat to being part of Birdy's waterpark experiences, so I swallowed my concerns and removed my cover-up. The insulin pump infusion set was stuck to the back of my right arm, the tubing snaking down my back a bit and was tucked into my bathing suit, insulin pump clipped to the back. My Dexcom sensor was inserted on my right thigh. Even though these devices are reasonably discreet, I felt like I had two giant toasters stuck to my body.

Birdy needed help climbing to a higher platform in the play area and I helped her do that. We ended up in the sprinkler pad for a while and I was thankful that the tape around my Dexcom sensor was strong enough to withstand the water. After a few minutes, I got over the whole "I don't want to wear giant toasters" feeling and got on with things.

"Excuse me. Is that an insulin pump?" All casual, the question came from behind me, where one of the park lifeguards was standing. His arms were crossed over his chest as he confidently watched the pool, but his question was quiet.

"Yeah, it is." I wasn't in the mood to have a full chat about diabetes, but I didn't want to make him feel awkward for asking.

"You like it?"

"I like it better than taking injections. I was diagnosed when I was a kid, so the pump is a nice change of pace from the syringes."

"I bet." He paused. "I was diagnosed last August and I've been thinking about a pump. But I hadn't ever seen one before. Is that it?" He pointed to the back of my arm.

"Kind of. That's where the insulin goes in, but the pump is this silver thing back here," I pointed to the back of my bathing suit, where my pump was clipped. "This is the actual pump. It's waterproof." A kid ran by, arms flailing and sending splashes of water all over the both of us.

"Good thing," he said.

"For real."

Birdy ran by to give me a high-five and then took off playing again.

"Your kid?"

"Yep."

"How long have you had diabetes?"

"Twenty-seven years."

He gave me a nod. "Thanks for not making it seem like it sucks. Enjoy your day," and he moved towards a group of kids that were playing a little roughly. I stayed and continued to watch my daughter play, very aware of my diabetes devices that, for the first time ever, didn't seem quite noticeable enough.

95

Diabetes Community

Diabetes Community

My first experience of a community of people with diabetes came from diabetes camp. I went to Clara Barton Camp as a child, and it was the first time I was surrounded by people with diabetes. All the campers had type 1 diabetes, as did the counselors, and even the majority of the staff had diabetes.

In the morning, they'd roll in this cart of insulin and syringes and all the campers would take their injections together. Essential drugs before breakfast. It was a rare moment, doing that as part of a group, being part of the majority.

Between camp life and access to the diabetes online community, there was a huge gap in access to other people living with diabetes. I felt alone, in a diabetes sense, during these years. That loneliness sucked.

Then I started blogging. Through the Internet, I met so many other people with diabetes. Because of blogging and the growing ecosystem of the digital diabetes community, there were structured events that brought people with diabetes together, as well as impromptu gatherings and community meet-ups.

Finding my community has made all the difference in my health and my emotional well-being. And yes, it is a little on the unusual side to share a bunch of personal health information online with strangers, but through those stories, we became friends. A family, of sorts. Which is a great by-product of a chronic illness.

The essays here are about how being part of the DOC (diabetes online community) has been crucial to my healthcare experience, and why watching it grow and change means so much to me.

People Who Need People

I first started blogging because I felt alone and wanted to find more than diabetes misery in my "diabetes" search returns on Google. That was five years ago. The blogosphere was shiny and new(ish, at least), and the diabetes blogosphere was in its infancy, with very few "real" voices carrying over the snake oil spammers and professional medical sites. Even though I had buddies from Clara Barton Camp and even though I knew of one or two other diabetics through friends of friends, I didn't have a network of people who really "got it."

But the Internet grew, and the diabetes community grew with it. Today we have hundreds of diabetes blogs and dozens of diabetes chat discussions on Twitter and Facebook groups and forums and Flickr groups and entire social networks and on and on and ... well, on.

Last night, during the #dsma (Diabetes Social Media Advocacy) discussion on Twitter, I realized that the shift is happening again. The discussion was turning towards how to help connect with other diabetics who weren't online and who didn't have access to the online community.

Before blogging, I was searching for online diabetes connections because there were very few people with diabetes in my offline life. I liked connecting with others online because I was sort of cloaked in the then-anonymity of the Internet. I could talk about the feelings stirred up by that nasty 242 mg/dl blood sugar the other morning, or the shame in skipping my workout so I could go out to dinner.

But after blogging about these experiences, I would log off and return to "real life," where no one knew much about what life was really like with diabetes.

Then the lines started to blur, and I wanted to remove that cloak.

I wanted to know more than just the diabetes sides of these people's personalities. In person meet ups were scheduled, and dinners started to become regular monthly events, and I started removing the caveat of "blogger" when I was referring to my new friends. Blog life and real life weren't as separate as they once were, and while diabetes was more of a discussion point than it had ever been before, it felt like a smaller part of my life. Love, marriage, friends, traveling, hobbies ... those things seem to take precedence over diabetes. While I still managed my condition closely, I felt like I could breathe easier, knowing there were all these people who really understood how I felt. And the more I got to know these people, the better I felt about my diabetes.

Which is why it makes perfect sense that people went online to find people they could hang out with in person. Full circle. We're just a bunch of people who need people.

I realized that even though the Internet provides so much support and information for people living with diabetes, there isn't anything quite like talking face-to-face with another person with diabetes. The words you speak out loud may be the very same ones you'd write in a blog post or comment, but there is something so cool about seeing the actual arched eyebrow or tugging grin or wild hand gesture. And as the diabetes community grows online, I see it budding and blooming in "real life," in meet ups and dinner dates and conferences.

Diabetes on your own can be a very heavy burden. Lots to manage, lots to juggle, and lots of emotions to muddle through at any given time. But with the kind of support that we, as members of this community have access to, it's like a helium injection.

And it all gets lighter, and easier to carry.

On Paper

"You write a blog about diabetes? Don't you run out of things to write about?"

A really nice lady at the JDRF event past weekend posed this question to me. I thought about it for a minute.

There's always something, some bit of minutiae to choose to chronicle. Maybe the blood sugar of 70 mg/dL coupled with a southeasterly Dexcom arrow that woke me up at 3 am. Could be the realization that I haven't changed my lancet in *mumble mumble* days. Or my husband's question – "Do we have AA batteries?" – and my immediate thought of "I use them in the pump. I hope we do!"

Could be that every meal, every snack, every bit of exercise, every time before I drive, every time I pee ("Is this high blood sugar or is this just ... the need to pee?") ... so many moments take something diabetes-related into account. It's not "woe is we" but sometimes just **whoa**, because diabetes can take up a lot of thought space.

"No, there's pretty much always something to write about," I answered.

And her face fell a little bit, and I realized she was asking not for herself, but for her son who was living with type 1 diabetes. I didn't realize that the underlying question wasn't about writing prompts but more, "Will diabetes always be on his mind?"

Diabetes will always be on his mind, just a little. Just enough to keep tabs on it. Sometimes more often, depending on the needs of his body and his mind.

But even though there will be so many moments when diabetes is taken into consideration throughout the course of our lives with it, they're just moments. They don't define his whole life.

"There's always something to write about, but I choose to write about these diabetes things and to focus on them." I amended, wanting to hug her. "I'm not highlighting these moments in my life ... just on paper."

She smiled, looking relieved. "They only take up so much room on screen, right?"

"Exactly," I said, bending the truth just enough to give her comfort.

Fine

"You have diabetes? You seem fine."

"I am fine."

On an average day, diabetes falls under the "annoying but tolerable" category. I test my blood sugar, wear any combination of continuous glucose monitoring device/insulin pump technology, do the insulin-to-carb math, eat decently, exercise as often and as hard as I can ... blah, blah, blaaaaaaaaah. For the most part, I don't see extreme hypoglycemia or excessive highs, and even though I see bits and pieces of diabetes in so many of my daily moments, it's not something that keeps me from pursuing the better parts of the day.

But on some days, diabetes falls into the "eff the effing islet you refused to ride in on" category.

Those are the days when my infusion set cannula kinks up underneath my skin and sends my blood sugar cruising into the 400's.

Or the days when a blood sugar of 38 mg/dL serves as a sweaty and panicked wake-up call at two in the morning. Or I let my brain wander around the fact that I've had this disease far longer than I'll ever have anything else, and I fear the impact of these fluctuating blood sugars on my quality of life, and longevity, going forward.

It's this weird dance, the one between feeling like diabetes profoundly affects my day-to-day health, both emotionally and physically, and the feeling that diabetes is just a blip on my daily radar.

"You seem fine."

I am fine. I think? I have a chronic illness - a disease - that compromises the function of my pancreas to the point where I need synthetic insulin daily, and even with dedicated management, I may see serious and debilitating complications in my lifetime. That's part of the dance, of feeling and *seeming* fine and actually *being* fine, even though my body is dealing with something serious every moment of every day.

Is it an invitation for a pity party? Nope. But it's a reminder that even though I feel fine, and I mostly am fine, there's a part of me that permanently needs tending to, and ignoring it only leads to tougher roads. The lows and the highs feel like they're ships passing by, but what they may be leaving in their wake scares me.

I don't live with any difficult diabetes complications at the moment (aside from closely-monitored and currently non-progressive retinopathy), and my A1C is at a comfortable constant, so diabetes does feel quiet and well-behaved at the moment, even after twenty-six years. But I know what it can do, and has done, and what it's capable of.

"I am fine."

It doesn't mean I want people to ignore the severity and pervasiveness of this disease. I don't want people who might be thinking about donating their time, energies, and finances to diabetes research, funding, and advocacy to be deterred by the fact that sometimes we look fine.

What those outside of this condition need to understand is that this perception of "fine" is all relative. One day you can be fine, and the next, things can be deeply and profoundly changed.

Sometimes diabetes will be in headlines, and on television shows, and health and mainstream media websites alike will turn their attention on the disease so many of us live with and care for every day. It's in those moments when we need to show the world that even though we seem fine, we still need better treatments and a cure for this disease.

Advocacy is important, and we can make a difference in diabetes in our lifetimes. Fine is status quo. Fine is living with insulin therapy. Fine is tolerating stereotypes instead of changing them. Fine is waiting patiently for things to change.

But we can do better.

Advice for Newbies

I feel weird giving advice because, even after 30 plus years of diabetes, I'm still trying to figure things out. Oftentimes, I'm still piecing together what feels like the right move, adding in uncertainty and trying to consider the concept of responsibility.

As much as it sucks sometimes, I have to be responsible. Some days that might mean sitting on the phone for hours trying to get through to my insurer. Other days it means moving finances around in order to make sure we have the bandwidth for my medical necessities. Every day it means taking my insulin, checking my blood sugar and caring about the results. As often as possible, I exercise and try to prioritize healthy foods with fewer carbs to minimize blood sugar spikes. I make myself follow through on doctor appointments and health check-ups. ... and occasionally, I go off the rails entirely with this whole responsibility thing and have a doughnut and sit on the couch and watch entire seasons of Game of Thrones but I think that comes back to responsibility in a roundabout way because you can't be game (of thrones) on all the time.

Mental health matters and my brain needs breathing room from the constant bitching and moaning from my pancreas.

My advice? Take this diabetes thing seriously. Even when it's hard. Diabetes can be a pain to deal with in some obvious ways, but it can concurrently ruin you with whispers, with signs and symptoms that aren't readily noticeable until something is very wrong.

It's much easier to respect the disease in efforts to earn the right to feel "fine." It's a weird road to walk, this one with diabetes, but you don't go it alone. (Need proof? Well, you have me, someone who has written about diabetes for almost twenty years. And if you click on any diabetes hashtag or campaign or Facebook page, etc. you'll find 10,000 other people ready to hold your hand and flip the middle finger to your pancreas at a moment's notice.)

Twice

"I have family members with diabetes, but they don't take care of themselves," he said.

"They eat whatever they want, and they never test their blood sugar, and they never go to the doctor."

The unspoken thought, capping the end of that sentence, is "... so they deserve whatever they get."

I had a hard time keeping my mouth shut, even though I was at this dinner with people I didn't really know, and who didn't really know me. They were aware of the fact that I have diabetes, but it wasn't a big discussion point throughout the day, so I think it was a little snippet of information that fell by the wayside by the time dinner was served.

"But how do you know that?" I blurted out.

He stopped and looked at me. "What do you mean?"

"How do you know they don't take care of themselves? Or go to the doctor? Or test their blood sugar?"

"Because they don't. I never see it. Not even at holidays."

I had zero desire to be the one who raises her voice at dinner table with strangers, preaching on about the misconception society has about diabetes, and about all the different kinds of people who live with it, etc. I wanted to have dinner, and hang out, and have a good time.

But I don't like the "yeah, but the majority of people with diabetes DON'T take care of themselves" argument, because I take care of myself. I try, and I do. And I know so many people who take care of themselves the best they can, and so many who, despite dedicated efforts, still run a rough road.

Perfection isn't achievable, and guilt is inescapable.

Chris encourages me to not take these kinds of discussions personally, because he hates to see my feelings seared, but it's hard not to take it personally. I have diabetes. They're talking about diabetes. Even when I try, it's hard to keep my views objective.

"Did you see me test my blood sugar at the table a few minutes ago?"

"You did?"

"Yeah. I have tested twice, actually, at this table. While you sat there. And that orange juice I had before? Which might not have seemed like the 'right' food for a diabetic? I was treating a low blood sugar. You don't always see what we do to take care of ourselves. But there's a lot that we do. I swear." I smiled at him, but inside I was pleading for him to see me as a person who, however my life wrings out, didn't deserve pain.

There was an awkward silence.

"Twice? You tested twice?"

"Yeah."

This time, erasing all awkwardness, he said, "Maybe they do stuff I don't see, too."

I beamed, wanting to jump across the table and hug him.

The Scaffolding

Who would be my biggest diabetes support?

Would it be my mom, who learned to pinch hit as my pancreas before I started second grade, making sure I had a childhood that wasn't owned by diabetes? Would it be my friends, who instinctively carry tubes of glucose tabs in their glove compartments or purses without even realizing it? Would it be my pediatric endocrinologist, who never forgot that liking boys and sleepovers at my best friend's house were just as important as blood sugar logs and insulin injections? Would it be this online community of fellow diabetics, who understand that there's a real life to be lived, even after diagnosis? Or would my hero be my husband, who has championed my health and made me feel like I was every bit the bride, no matter what the status of my pancreas?

There are so many people who are part of my life with diabetes. But life is more than all this diabetes stuff. Diabetes doesn't define me. It doesn't define my relationships, either.

In my head, diabetes is just one part of the core of who I am. And the people who support me, and my diabetes "stuff," are part of the scaffolding that keeps me steady. Diabetes is a constant in my life, but also a constantly shifting priority. Some days, I don't need much help or care and diabetes maintenance is on the back burner of my life.

Other days, it's a huge part of the day and requires a lot of attention. And then there are the in between days. Regardless of how loudly diabetes is fussing on any given day, the people in my life who support me aren't viewing my health as a project we need to constantly discuss or assess. It's what we do, as a family, almost without thinking.

Those people I mentioned - my parents, my husband, my friends, my medical team, and you, dear readers - are the permanent scaffolding in my life. The structure that I almost forget is there sometimes, because it's folded so seamlessly around the rest of my life. You all help me repair and maintain my health, wrapping neatly around the whole of me and keeping me standing tall and strong.

On the easier days, I take it a bit for granted.

But on the hard days, I'm able to stand tall, thanks to this support.

Diabetes Club*

1st Rule: You do NOT talk about diabetes.
2nd Rule: … just kidding, of course you can talk about diabetes.
3rd Rule: If someone says "I'm low" or goes limp, grab some glucose tabs.
4th Rule: Only two CGM transmitters to an order.
5th Rule: One snack at a time.
6th Rule: No insulin, no bolus.
7th Rule: Diabetes will go on as long as you go on.
8th Rule: If this is your first time at diabetes, you have to diabetes. But you won't go it alone.

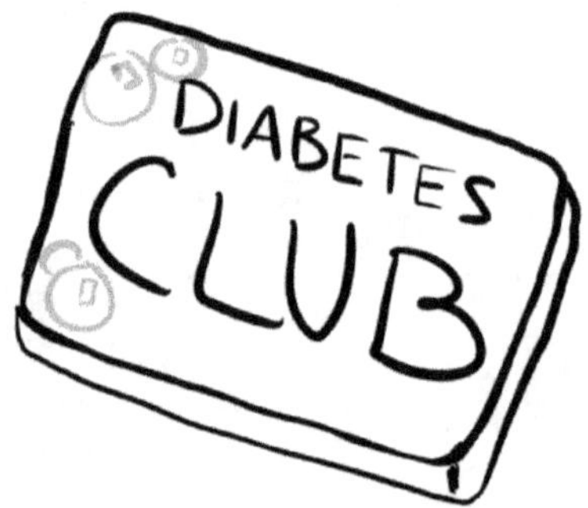

** in homage to the rules of Fight Club. I mean, some club. That we don't talk about. Shhhh. And yes, there are several Fight Club references in this book.*

Joslin Medalists: How Far We've Come, and How Far We Can Go

During the Joslin medalist meeting last week, I didn't say anything. I wasn't presenting or doing any kind of networking. I was invited as "media" (totally in quotes) but I attended as a grown-up child with diabetes, hoping to continue on that path of growing up.

I sat next to a woman named Eleanor (my beloved grandmother's name) and she had been living with type 1 for 58 years. She asked to see pictures of my daughter. She offered me a cough drop after I spent a few minutes trying to clear my throat, and she stuck her hand out to take the wrapper, spying my pump tubing jutting out from my pocket. "I don't wear a pump," she said. "I do just fine with my needles. And you appear to be doing just fine with your pump. Do you need another cough drop?"

As Dr. George King, director of research at the Joslin Clinic, gave his opening remarks, quotes from the medalists were flashing up on the screen behind him. "I have learned to understand that perfection is not possible." "Tomorrow is another chance to do better." "Say YES to every opportunity."

These people were incredible because of what they've accomplished with type 1 diabetes. Hilary Keenan, PhD and pat of the Joslin biostatistics team, stunned me with the stats on this group. Their average A1C is 7.3%, with an average diagnosis age of 11 years old. Their average age is 70. The average duration of their diabetes is 59 years. The most common ages for their type 1 diagnosis are age 6 and age 12. And this group of medalists have a very low rate of proliferative retinopathy and kidney disease.

I sat in this room, listening intently, and thinking about my own life. I've had diabetes for 24 years. Long enough to appreciate where I've come from and what I've accomplished, and yet still a rookie in the eyes of these medalists.

Not only are they brilliantly healthy, despite their diabetes, but they're also insightful and wise in that way that only decades of life can bring. They stood up, one at a time, and introduced themselves to the group. Their stories made me laugh out loud (like when the lady was talking about her CGM and her pump, and then someone's phone rang and she stopped to ask, "What kind of meter is that?" and the other woman answered, "It's a phone?"), made me grateful, and made me cry openly in this room of strangers.

"Eliot Joslin was my first endocrinologist. He wore a charcoal gray suit and a crisp white shirt. And the first time I met with him I said, 'Oh my God, he's an undertaker!'"

"Diabetes has given me so many opportunities. I had a chance to spend time with Bret Michaels." Pause. "But I didn't know who he was. Now I do, though!"

"I have seen many doctors retire. I don't have that option, so I keep finding new doctors."

One man talked about the party he threw for himself when he reached 63 years with type 1, as part of his 70th birthday party. "I handed out certificates to the people who helped me get here. And I had one for Eliot Joslin that said, 'Helped to keep me alive, despite myself.'"

"We do our best. And to God trust the balance."

"I was diagnosed when I was one. My doctors told my parents I would die in my early 20's. My parents didn't tell me this until I was, oh, well into my 50's."

"I'm here today, really, because of my wife," said a man with shaking hands.

"Today, I brought with me my beautiful daughter. Her name is Joslin. I named her for this wonderful place."

But one man broke my heart entirely when he quietly stood up and addressed the group of his peers, his fellow people with diabetes with more than 50 years under their belt.

"One year, I asked the woman behind the counter how many of us there were. How many medalists? And she said that out of the million and a half type 1 diabetics, only about 1000 survive 50 years. And it wasn't until I was driving home that I realized what we're up against." He paused and put his hand to his collar, absently touching the ribbon on his medal. "And that is when I cried."

This whole experience was so inspiring, so humbling, and made me so aware of what diabetes has the potential to affect in my life. I was born decades after these people were diagnosed, so I know things have changed for the better, as far as treatment options. I know the outcome for people living with type 1 diabetes has improved by leaps and bounds.

This group of medalists began their journey with glass syringes and twice-yearly finger sticks. We are a new generation of people with diabetes, and we put our hope on the foundations built by the medalists before us.

Ordinary but Extraordinary

I will admit right here, right now that I admire people who accomplish incredible physical feats while also doing the whole diabetes thing. Climbing Everest? Hell yes! Ultramarathon? Hell yes! Hang-gliding across Iceland while knitting a sweater onto your body as it hang-glides? Hell to the absolute yes – and why hasn't anyone tried this?

I'll also admit right here, right now that I may never be one of those Everest climbing, ultramarathon'ing, hang-glide-knitter PWDs. Not because I can't or shouldn't but because my goals don't battle out in that arena. And that's okay.

Sometimes the inspiration I'm searching for doesn't come from the big, incredible-feat stories. They inspire me like whoa, but not as much when I was sitting looking at my stupid CGM graph that was frustratingly elevated while traveling yesterday. I needed someone to post a crappy CGM graph at that moment, so I could see that I wasn't the only one not rocking "perfect" blood sugars, and that I could also regroup and move on.

I mean, I know I can regroup and move on. But it's nice to see your own struggles/successes reflected in the stories from others.

The inspiration that I benefit from daily comes through social media, via ordinary, everyday stuff. These folks aren't necessarily posting photos of their pump sites from the top of a mountain (although some do), but are showing their regular lives with diabetes.

What they've overcome that day might have been an insurance battle. Or they finally paid off a medical bill that's been causing stress for months. They might be snuggling their baby, who may have been marked as an impossible dream. Putting in a pump site on their arm for the first time.

They might have just crossed the finish line on their first 5k, or gone for a run for the first time in their life, or went for a walk around their office building on a lunch break, making time for exercise even during the work day because they are worth it.

Ordinary as can be! And yet heroic, to me.

It's parents of kids with diabetes shouldering the burden of the disease so their kid can roll through their childhood as unaffected as possible. It's the adults with diabetes fighting back against societal stereotypes and insurance denials and insulin access issues. It's the voices of people with type 2, who remain the majority of PWD but are woefully underrepresented in the online community.

There are so many "small stories" that are making big differences, and I wish they were perceived as sexy/aspirational/inspirational as summiting a mountain.

I'm sometimes daunted by the Big Things being accomplished at times, wondering where smaller stories fit into the narrative of diabetes.

Like, am I weird if I feel accomplished for renewing all my prescriptions? Or from losing 4 lbs of relentless baby weight by way of just walking? The small victories seem so small sometimes, especially on days when diabetes lives a little large, but they remain victories nonetheless.

Props to everyone who is doing something powerfully positive with diabetes ... like living with it. Whether that's climbing a mountain. Or raising a family. Or hang-gliding across Iceland while knitting that sweater onto your body as you hang-glide around.

Or making toast.

These stories – all of them – show diabetes in the context of real life. And all of these stories are inspiring in their own way.

It's not about attention. Or accolade. Or high-fives for big deal things. It's about looking at how diabetes is presented and seeing your story – the good, the bad, and the ugly – represented.

The Quiet Parts

Despite having shared so much of my diabetes thoughts and experiences through my blog, you might think that there aren't any topics I'm unwilling to tackle. But there are plenty of things I have decided not to share, both in the realm of diabetes and in the regular flow of insulin-free life. I'm an oddly private person, considering how much I like to share (sometimes awkward) stories. What do I share, and what do I choose not to share, and why?

"You put it out there [on the Internet], so you're inviting people to judge you."

That's true. By putting our lives "out there," we are giving people information to judge us, for better or for worse. Giving the specifics of my lab work results or my weight or my fasting blood sugar this morning provides people with a window into my health reality. It lets people think of me as little more than a statistic, or a range, or an assumption. Some people are comfortable with allowing that kind of access. I have come to realize that I'm not that kind of person.

No, I won't tell you my A1C, even if it's stellar and in-range and covered in glitter. I work very hard to manage this disease, and I've come to realize that I'm not the kind of person who does well being judged for that specific number, especially when that judgment attempts to minimize my efforts.

Because I cared very much about the critique for a few years. There was a time when I posted about my A1C while preparing for pregnancy (it was higher than what my doctor recommended, and I was writing about my struggle in bringing it down to baby range), and the comments that came back about my number ranged in their tone and sentiment. Invited, warranted, or not, I can handle critical commentary, but there is a fine line between "constructive criticism" and "cruelty."

And once I stopped getting all twitchy about the unsupportive commentary - because it's not all going to be supportive - I felt a lot better. Getting older has made me care less about being judged and more comfortable and confident about my decisions, decisions like not sharing my personal lab data. Or like decisions to write about diabetes, online or otherwise, in the first place.

"Just because you give them a window doesn't mean you have to give them a door."

We are not obligated to share. We chose to share. I wrote a website and this book, and will continue to write as ideas move me, because of the connection to the diabetes community that sharing fosters. I love that part of it. It took me a long time to realize where my boundaries are, and to feel comfortable staying within them.

While I chronicled my pregnancy in a very detailed way, I didn't share everything. Before my daughter was even born, I decided to keep her name offline, and after sharing some of her baby stories, I decided to keep her offline, too. And I share a lot of the silly things related to diabetes, and some of the complicated things, too, but there are thoughts I have about diabetes that are sometimes so terrifying and other times so arrogant that I keep those in, too.

Diabetes is so personal and runs every kind of gamut. Sharing it all feels like too much, at times. Sharing some, however, helps me deal with the emotional side of this chronic illness.

A window in our lives? That sounds nice. Opening the door and letting in everything, and everyone? I can't manage that kind of flow. What if a bat flies into my living room? Fuck bats. So I'm sticking with the windows, with the screens and screening tools firmly in place.

"What kinds of stories will we never hear you tell? And why won't you tell them?"

I don't share stories about my extended family without their permission. I don't post about where I live or where I work during the day. I absolutely do not write about arguments with family. I do not share things that make me sad while I'm going through them (but sometimes I will share once I'm on the other side of that kind of emotional upheaval, as is my comfort level).

This kind of paints life as though it might be going well all the time and without struggle, but I think we all know that the stuff we read on the Internet and writ large is always written with specific bias and through a specific lens. (Though I do try to disclose my financial biases, and also, I will always like my kids more than I like your kid. It's a fact. Unless you are my husband, in which case I like your kids as much as I like my kids, for obvious reasons.)

I won't tell some of these stories because they sometimes hurt to go through, never mind the added pain of retelling them. I won't tell them because they are mine, and privacy is an often-underrated but essential part of a peaceful life.

What I will share are stories about how diabetes affects my life, and how it plays a part in shaping my experiences. I will connect with others through these stories and those friendships will color my existence in a way that I am still understanding and always appreciating. I will share in hopes that someone will feel less alone, just like I feel less alone every time I read a new diabetes writer or have an awkward interaction with someone in a bathroom.

Regardless of how much or how little you share, your voice is important, and our community flourishes as a result.

Mentalbetes

Mentalbetes

My six-year-old son and I were listening to music the other day, and he was confused about why people write so many sad songs.

"Do they like feeling sad? Why do they write about feeling sad?"

"Sometimes people write about their emotions in order to process how they feel. I do that with my diabetes emotions sometimes. I do it with other emotions, too. Writing helps me figure out how I'm feeling."

"It helps you know how you feel?" Short pause while he thought it through. "Like you didn't know how you felt before you started writing?"

"Sometimes. Putting the words down on paper helps make things clearer for me."

Clinicians, researchers, and people living with diabetes alike talk about diabetes in very binary ways, focusing on A1Cs and carb ratios and the math portions of this illness.

But after 36 years with diabetes, I've found that the emotions are wound tightly around life with chronic illness, and they need as much tending to as any glucose meter result. No doubt that numbers require wrangling, but it helps to have your mental state in order because it makes doing the diabetes to-dos easier. Much easier to make self-care and healthcare a priority when you are feeling emotionally healthy.

Writing about these feelings has helped me work through them. Finding words to describe the mental load of diabetes adds clarity. The essays in this section of the book are all about that mental load, and efforts to make it feel lighter.

Define or Explain

"Diabetes doesn't define you; it just helps explain you."

It struck me that he was right.

My brother and I don't talk about diabetes very much. I don't remember ever talking about it when we were kids. We played with Legos and built army forts for the hamsters to live in. There weren't any big diabetes discussions and, quite frankly, we never really talked about it until I started my diabetes-centric blog.

But during a discussion we had today, it came up.

"Diabetes doesn't define you; it just helps explain you."

Diabetes didn't make me smart, but being regimented and dedicated to achieving results on a medical level may have made me work harder in school. Diabetes didn't make me determined, but it may have contributed to my constant drive towards my ever-changing definition of success.

Such perspective is gained from a chronic condition, regardless of its complications. It doesn't define me, but the strongest parts of my personality may have been gently shaped by the perspective gained from having it.

Diabetes didn't make me love with such ease, but having tasted my own mortality makes every hug, every laugh, every kiss that much more needed and appreciated.

I hope so fiercely for a cure. I hope for a cure every time I see a press release about new research breakthroughs. I hope every time I test my blood sugar that the numbers will always be in range. I hope every time I go to Joslin. I hope every day.

"Diabetes doesn't define you; it just helps explain you."

I didn't ask what he meant because I already knew. Diabetes isn't the whole of me. It doesn't own me or define me or ruin me. He and I both know that.

When I wake up every morning and test my blood sugar, when I prime the pump with insulin, when I calculate the carbohydrates in a meal, I know it doesn't define me. But when I am feeling anxious or scared about my medical future or just simply overwhelmed, I know it doesn't define me.

It just helps explain me.

What's it like to take insulin?

The act of inserting the needle is one thing. Years ago, I drew insulin into a syringe from a vial, tapping out the bubbles and then pressing the needle tip to my skin. Thirty years ago, my style was to press the needle through my skin in a slow, deliberate sort of manner, using the speed to gauge whether or not the injection site would hurt (and if it felt uncomfortable at first press, I'd move to a different place). I still do it this way now, whether it's a syringe, an insulin pen, or the infusion set for my insulin pump. Controlling the pain is important to me. It's on the short list of things I can control.

The kind of insulin has changed for me throughout the years, as well. Upon diagnosis in 1986, I took Regular and NPH, which were pretty sluggish and forced me to plan my meals around my morning insulin injection. I've also used Lente, Ultra Lente, Lantus, Levemir, Tresiba, Humalog, and Novolog. NPH used to be rolled in my mother's hands so it would mix properly before injection. Lantus burned when I took it, and the burn would spread under the injection site for a second or two. I'm currently using Humalog in my pump. It claims to start working in 15 minutes but my body seems to make that timeline 35 min.

Insulin is serious stuff. It lowers blood sugars. Not enough keeps blood glucose levels higher than is safe, subjecting my body to the abuses of elevated sugars. Too much insulin throws me into a "hypoglycemic event." I've had a number of low blood sugar episodes that have scared me. "Scared me" isn't really a fair description, either, because in some of those moments, I wondered if I was going to die. Not being dramatic, but more pragmatic. Will I be able to consume enough glucose to keep me from passing out, going into a coma, dying? These thoughts sometimes go through my mind like a stock market ticker tape when I'm severely hypoglycemic.

Physically, aside from putting a needle into my body, insulin is crucial to my body's metabolic processes. I'd be dead without it. Dead. It keeps my body from starving to death.

Acknowledging that is crazy, and gives way to the other side of taking insulin: the headspace side.

Acknowledging that my ability to stay alive relies on the contents of a small, glass vial is humbling as hell. The fact that so many people with diabetes cannot afford or access insulin and they die without it is beyond humbling. Every time I finish a bottle of insulin, I make sure to grab every last bit, waiting for any bubbles to burst and grabbing them when they go liquid. I do not waste insulin. A bottle broken against bathroom tile is mourned. And as the price of insulin continues to climb, my panic response does as well because not having insulin is not an option if I want to continue to exist.

That's some crazy shit to think about as I tap the bubbles from a syringe.

What's it like to take insulin? Humbling, if I think about how lucky I am to be alive after Banting and Best worked their science magic.

But the weird thing is, on most days, I don't think about it. This hormone I'd die without, this item in my fridge that's worth more than my entire house in total, it's not something I deliberate or celebrate every day. I just take it, ignoring any quick pinch on my skin and moving on.

And that right there illustrates how lucky I am.

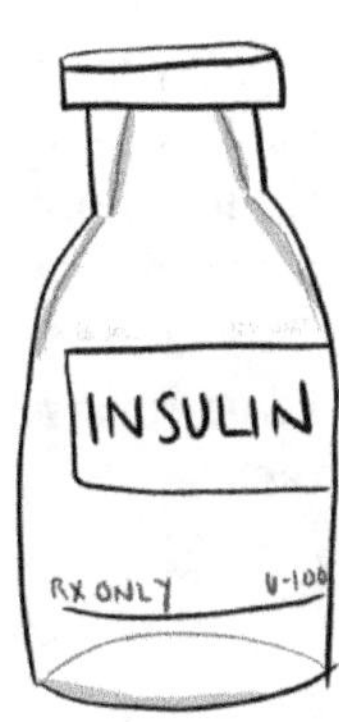

Duck on a Pond

I read an article about diabetes, and this quote gave me pause: "She said her mom equates living with diabetes to being 'like a duck on a pond: it looks graceful and calm just swimming along, but below the surface, you don't see the paddling, and all the work it's doing to keep moving forward." [1]

What would it be like to not be paddling so furiously? I tried to give that thought pattern a go.

I pictured waking up in the morning and leaning into the baby's crib to give him a smooch, then rubbing the sleep from my eyes while shuffling into the bathroom to brush my teeth. No checking my Dexcom graph immediately upon waking, no pricking my finger and challenging myself to put toothpaste on the toothbrush before the result comes up on the glucose meter.

I would put the little Guy on my hip and go wake up Birdy, not worrying if I was impaling my son's butt cheek on my insulin pump. No low blood sugar would keep me from bringing my kids downstairs in time to eat breakfast before the school bus came roaring by.

Super wet diapers or requests for more than one glass of water at dinner would not make my stomach drop and my heart feel heavy.

My day would consist of emails that had nothing to do with diabetes and video calls where I didn't keep a juice box just out of sight. I'd breastfeed my son without concerns about going low afterwards.

I'd go for a run with only my car keys and my phone – no glucose tabs.

Lunch would be a meal instead of a math problem (If my blood sugar is 103 mg/dL and I'm eating 15 grams of carbs and I pre-bolus 1u of insulin, will two trains leaving at the same time from Providence have enough glucose tabs on board to bring me up, should I start to tumble?). I'd plan my meals around what people wanted to eat and when they wanted to eat it.

I'd think Steel Magnolias was a really sad movie and that Sally Field is a tremendous actress instead of wondering for decades if Shelby was going to be me.

My body would be absent the scaly, itchy rash that comes up as a result of my diabetes device adhesive allergy. My fingertips would be smooth and unblemished. If I had a brief millisecond of clouded vision, I'd think, "Meh – something in my eye," instead of "DO I HAVE DIABETES IN MY EYE?!"

I would think dresses with pockets are cool instead of finding a cute dress with pockets and buying that same dress in every frigging color available.

I'd only have one pump – just the breast one - at my house.

Bank account balances would ebb and flow as a result of non-diabetes purchases and responsibilities, without that nagging need to have a clot of cash for constant copays, premiums, and out-of-pocket medical expenses. That need for medical insurance would be a source of stress but not a boiling point of panic.

I'd see cupcakes and giggle about how they're "diabetes on a plate," blissfully unaware of how fucking ignorant "diabetes on a plate" sounds.

I'd worry about the future like everyone else instead of worrying like everyone else and then adding the un-scratchable itch to have three month's worth of insulin and syringes in my house at all times.

I'd fall asleep at night and expect to wake up in the morning, without issue.

I'd have a family and friends and would travel and write and experience things that are scary and exciting and a mush of both ...

... wait a fucking second. I have a family and friends. And I travel. And write. And I experience things that are scary and exciting and a mush of both. Diabetes does not keep me from living the life I want. It's an enormous pain in the ass at times and I have uneasy feelings about what it will look and feel like twenty years from now, but I am still here.

Imagining life without diabetes sounds nice and I can't wait to find out what it will be like. But I'm holding my own either way. Paddling on.

1. https://www.peoplenewspapers.com/2017/02/02/imagining-life-diabetes-free/

Sick Your Whole Life

Yesterday, I was at a meeting where the audience was decidedly not a diabetes one. And in explaining my experiences with diabetes, I had to give an overview of what type 1 diabetes is and how long I've been living with it.

"I was diagnosed at the age of seven. It will be 32 years this September ..."

After the presentation, an attendee approached me. "So you've been sick your whole life?"

The phrasing caught me off guard.

I don't think I've ever considered myself "sick." Diabetes is a disease and I understand the denotation and range of connotations of that word, but "sick" struck me in a strange way.

I feel sick when I have a cold. When I had pneumonia in college. That time I threw up in my purse. Whenever my previously-injured cornea flares up again. Stuff like that. Diabetes doesn't make me feel like I'm sick. Maybe it's because it's always been the constant, the thing that has always been the health issue on tap so much so that it has become part of the established background noise.

Or maybe because it's been relatively quiet as a disease, especially when I consider what it's capable of accomplishing.

Checking blood sugars? Taking insulin? I don't feel sick. Even when I'm really low or naggingly high, I don't feel sick, exactly. Those moments are rotten but they have passed so far. There's a strange barrier that I've put up, mentally, between the diabetes stuff and the "real people sick" sort of stuff.

"I've had diabetes for most of my life, yes." I said, letting the different connotations of "sick" linger a little longer, uneasy about what may come, unsure if I'll make room for that word.

Complicated

A few weeks ago, I was diagnosed with macular edema.

It's a complication you can't see, one that I can't see until I can't see. Sophisticated computer equipment and camera technology have afforded me the opportunity to find out early, giving me the chance to track this issue closely and opt for aggressive treatment options (laser surgery, medicated eye drops, intra-ocular steroid injections) when the time comes. I feel raw and vulnerable, but I have information. I have access to excellent doctors and specialists. I have options.

I also have a bit of a stomach ache because when I asked, "How can I keep this from becoming more of an issue, going forward?" the response was, "Keep your glucose control as close to 'normal' as possible."

It's the "as possible" bit that throws me.

It could have been the birthday cake?

It could have been the cupcakes I snuck, and lied about, as a kid?

It could have been NPH and Regular and hormones and the "brittle diabetes" moniker that they wrote in marker on my chart at the hospital made "normal" a definition built on shifting sand?

It could have been the pregnancy hormones, or the period of diabetes burnout I experienced after my daughter was born?

It could have been anything. Everything. It could have been the years of struggling. It could have been the quick transition to tight control. It could have been bad genes, or good genes, or tight jeans. It could have been everything I did, or didn't do.

The truth is, it was type 1 diabetes.

We don't talk about complications often in this community, and I hope that's because many people aren't dealing with them. Discussions about "what could happen" are often left in those quotation marks, as if that holds the threat captive.

But after decades with type 1 diabetes, complications may happen. Retinopathy, kidney issues, depression ... the list is long and a good attitude, a determined mind, and even good control don't keep these issues entirely at bay. I've had my share of issues with my eyes. In the past, I've seen some cotton wool spots in my eyes. And during the course of my pregnancy, retinopathy near the macula dictated a c-section delivery for my daughter. And now, this diagnosis of macular edema in my right eye.

This doesn't mean I've failed.

I am sharing this because it's real life with diabetes. This is what's happening, and even though I don't want people thinking that diabetes complications are necessarily a guarantee, they also aren't a mark of failure. I work hard to manage this disease. I will keep trying, even though I know there will be more radar blips, and more moments that cause momentary tears but then renewed determination.

There's so much personal responsibility, so many moments of, "Well, you have the tools to manage this disease, so why aren't you hitting the mark?" Diabetes is unique, in that way, with complications often viewed as a result of the patient not working hard enough, when in fact, they are the result of diabetes.

By writing this, I'm opening myself up to people who want to point fingers and to say, "Well, it won't be my kid" or "It won't be me." I can understand that. I didn't think it would be me. I hope it's not you. But it might be you, and in the event that it is, I want you to know that you aren't alone. Diabetes complications need to be talked about, because the guilt that comes with their diagnosis can be crippling, melting away the value of our efforts.

It's easy to become overwhelmed when diabetes seems to be the leading cause of leading causes. For me, the diagnosis of macular edema made me want to wallow in self-pity for a while and hate diabetes, and I did that for a few days. I cried a little. I combed through internet search returns. I hugged my husband and my daughter, burying my face in the chaos of her pigtails and inhaling the scent of unconditional love (and baby shampoo). I called my mom. I talked with a few friends.

And then I moved on, because if I stay in that pool of guilt, I'll drown.

Guilt is a misplaced emotion when it comes to diabetes, and to related complications. It's not my fault that I have diabetes. It's not my fault that I have eye complications. But it is my job to take care of these issues, and to work through the moments where I want to give up. The guilt gnaws but I can't let it take too deep of a bite; I owe myself more than that. The emotional ebb and flow of diabetes has more impact on my happiness than the actual fluctuations of my blood sugars, so I won't be beating myself up about this. But, as I write some of this, I'm alternating between hitting keys and wiping tears angrily off my face, which pisses me off because even when I make a conscious decision to block feeling bad and guilty about it, I'm still unnerved. I want to be tough, but I'm not as good at that as I'd like to be. I want to be strong for my family, but sometimes I need them to be strong for me, in the moments when I'm buckling a little.

So they checked the box, the one that says, "Complicated." But I knew that, far before it was seen in my eyes. Life with diabetes is complicated. Life without it is pretty damn complicated, all on its own. But it's mine, this life, and it's still good. When I come to the end of the very last day, I want to feel happy. That's more my goal than an A1C number ever was, or ever will be.

Life moves forward, complicated as it may be.

Progress

"Everything looks good. No progress is good, actually. Means your eyes haven't deteriorated any further in the last five months." Dr S, my eye doctor at the Joslin Clinic, ran her fingers across the keyboard, typing notes into my online file.

"So it's the same as back in November? When I moved from mild to moderate retinopathy?"

"Right. Still non-proliferative, but the same. Not worse, by any stretch. We're working with a few spots, a very small bit of leakage, but nothing I'd recommend treatment for, other than watching it closely."

I let out the breath I didn't realize I was holding. The fluorescent bulbs in the room were bright and ricocheting off the white walls, making me feel like I was in an avalanche of light.

"We do want to check on one thing, though." She turned her chair towards me. "There appears to be some swelling of the optic nerve. And I'd like to have that checked more precisely with the OCT test."

I looked over at the eye chart on the far wall. When I had first come into the room, I wanted to go over to the teeniest line and commit it to memory, so I could recite it at will. "SNDRZ," I'd say, and they'd cancel all other tests that day, in recognition of my clever eyeballs.

"Okay. Was there swelling last time?" I couldn't remember it being mentioned.

"Yes, it's here in your chart. And from what I can tell, it's still present. But my measurements are subjective, and I'd like to run a more precise test, so we know exactly where we're at with this. The test is really just another picture of your eye; it's not painful."

"I can't argue with that. So sure, let's do that test."

I went back into the dilation waiting room to be called in for the OCT test. The lights were dim and a large television displayed HD images of starfish regenerating lost limbs as they crept along the ocean floor.

"The starfish reaches out with the limb that is still growing back. It remembers what was once there and what will be there again," Leonard Nimoy narrated. I pictured my eyeball, crawling across the ocean floor, trailing its optic nerve in the sand.

"Kerri Sparling?" The eye photographer (what is his official title?) brought me into a room. "Just rest your chin here, and stare straight ahead at the X. I'll tell you when you can blink, and we'll grab a few images of those eyes, okay?"

"Just look at the Space Invader thing in there?"

He laughed. "Yup, right at him." The OCT test was completed in a matter of quick clicks, and I returned to the waiting room to wait patiently for my doctor to review the results with me.

"Kerri? Come on back," Dr. S said, holding computer print outs in her hand. The office door shut with a snap, and we stood in the middle of the room, crowding around these papers like kids with a treasure map.

"This? Is your optic nerve. See how it's thick on both sides and has that dip in the middle?" She pointed, and I panicked.

"Should it have that!?"

"Yes, it's exactly what it should have. There isn't much swelling at all. Actually, there's barely any, which is why I wanted you to have this test in the first place, so we were measuring precisely and not panicking preemptively." She smiled warmly. "Everything looks good. Let's get together again in four months, okay?"

"Sounds great." I went to get the door, but turned back to her. "So my eyes are okay? I mean, not perfect and they still have the moderate retinopathy and all that crap, but there's nothing to panic about, right? I can hold steady and relax about this a little? You said no progress is a good thing, right? I tend to freak out. Does it show? I bet it shows," the incessant questions spilling from my mouth and my freakishly-dilated eyes..

"You are fine. Go home and enjoy that first birthday party. I'll see you in four months."

These appointments are hard for me to follow through on, for a dozen different reasons. But one of the big reasons is fear.

Sometimes I want to go full-on ostrich about this whole disease and pretend it's not happening. Weird thing is, I always feel better after I know where things stand. Even if the news isn't always the best news. I'm learning to roll with it.

And that's progress.

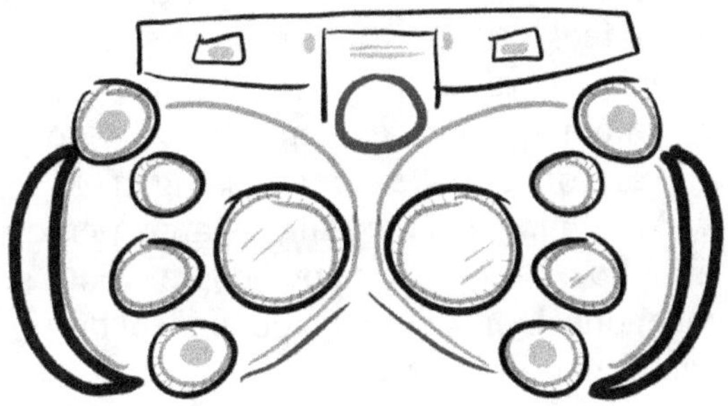

Filling Back Up

It whispered in my ear two Januarys ago, when a low blood sugar came too close to becoming terrifying as I felt the whoosh of that bullet go by. I'd never felt anything like that before, that aftermath of fear and numbness. Then I marked twenty-six years with type 1 diabetes, and I just wanted to outrun this disease, to stay ahead of it, to pretend that it can't ever possibly catch me.

Then there was this weird feeling, one I've never felt before. It wasn't depression, I don't think, because it didn't feel ... I don't know ... like anything I'd ever read about or been warned about by my doctor. I didn't feel uncontrollably sad, and I didn't have thoughts that would have concerned my family.

There was this emptiness, though. I can't put my finger on where it came from or what its role was in my life. Not an all-consuming feeling, but it did strike me at the oddest times, like during a conference when I was hoping to be more social, or during a movie that was supposed to make me laugh, or like when I would be in the car by myself and pull into the driveway of my house, and I'd feel lost. And empty. Coming into the house and seeing my happy daughter and my husband filled me back up, but for those brief moments before opening the car door and letting the sounds from outside come rushing in, the quiet was overwhelming. I'm normally a happy person – quick to laugh, and happy to be surrounded by people – but I suddenly wanted to be alone, only being alone made me feel better, for a few minutes, then ultimately worse.

I talked with some people, including my husband and my closest friends, trying to understand why I felt this way and how to keep the feelings from becoming dominant. It wasn't all diabetes-related, but there was something about having had this disease for twenty-six years that made me feel trapped. I started doing destructive math in my head, about how nothing had been introduced into my life that I'd had longer than type 1 diabetes.

Diabetes has been part of my life for longer than school, longer than any romantic relationship, longer than any hobby, longer than any car or t-shirt or memory. I thought about life's milestones and the influence of diabetes on each one, sometimes just a light touch, not enough to leave the smallest mark, other times a heavy-handed drag of claws.

A few months after marking the twenty-sixth anniversary of my diagnosis, I turned 34 years old and felt convinced that I was having a mid-life crisis. I feared death, actively and aggressively, nervous to go to sleep at night because of the low blood sugars that crept in. I started feeling nervous about unreasonable things. Panic attacks, like the ones I had back in college (when my parents split and my immediate family life was very unsettled) revisited for a few weeks, making my chest feel tight and making me wonder if it was panic or was I having a years-of-type-1-diabetes-induced heart attack.

While marking a diabetes anniversary was the catalyst for darker times, acknowledging the feelings that made me feel unsettled made healing easier.

I didn't see a therapist (though I would if these feelings were to resurface) and I didn't add medications to my list (though I would have, were they necessary), but I did ease myself into things like family trips, private (non-blog) journaling, and finding time to dedicate to quiet jogs that stopped my brain from going into panicky overdrive.

I started filling back up, emotionally.

One afternoon, I realized it had been days since I'd felt empty. Weeks went by, turning into months, and then the emptiness started to become harder to remember, harder to pinpoint the "why" of, and life felt more like I remembered before my twenty-sixth diabetes anniversary.

I don't miss feeling that way – all that emptiness – but I'm not surprised that I felt it. Diabetes is intrusive and touches everything, like a kid with grubby hands. For decades, I didn't mind wiping away the fingerprints that were left everywhere, but last year, I reached not so much a breaking point, but a moment when I couldn't bend things any further without snapping.

I didn't want to deal with this disease. I was mad. Overwhelmed. And then that empty. It was a strange grieving process for a disease that wasn't going anywhere and for a life that wasn't over.

It was raining a little when I started running this past Tuesday morning, September 10th, but I decided to go anyway. I set out after sticking my running belt underneath my shirt instead of over it, to protect the Dexcom receiver from the rain. Sneakers worn from a year's worth of logging miles and my pump clipped to the top of my pants, I ran.

I'm not a pretty runner – I slog and huff and puff and probably resemble more 'laboring pug' than 'actual human' while I'm on the trail, but I made the decision to keep going. With each step, it didn't get easier. I wasn't riding endorphins during my run, and I felt the strain on my muscles and my resolve, but I kept going because it's good for me to run. It's good for me to try. It's good to feel healthy and to look healthy and to be healthy.

The following day, Wednesday the 11th, I marked my twenty-seventh anniversary with type 1 diabetes.

I wish I had a more gracious outlook on my experiences with diabetes, but I don't. I wish I felt that it was some kind of blessing, but to me, it isn't. It's a thorn in my side that digs in deeper with every passing anniversary, but fuck you, diabetes.

I'm tired at times, but I'm not stopping. I'm afraid, but I'm still going.

Diabetes has brought me to some of the edges of life, daring me to look into the abyss and wonder just how long I'd know I was falling before I hit the ground, but there's power in that. I'm living with diabetes, with all the accompanying ugliness and arrogance, power and determination, all the perspective and perseverance and bitterness, all the fear and fearlessness that comes with any life, but is micro-scoped and magnified by a disease that never, ever takes a breath and doesn't leave my world until I do.

Yesterday, my daughter and I baked a cake, but I didn't eat it, or explain why or why not. She wanted to make a fancy treat, and I wanted to see her smile.

We put candles on it, hummed a sort of tuneless 'happy birthday,' and blew them out, marking a celebration of absolutely nothing and at the same time, everything.

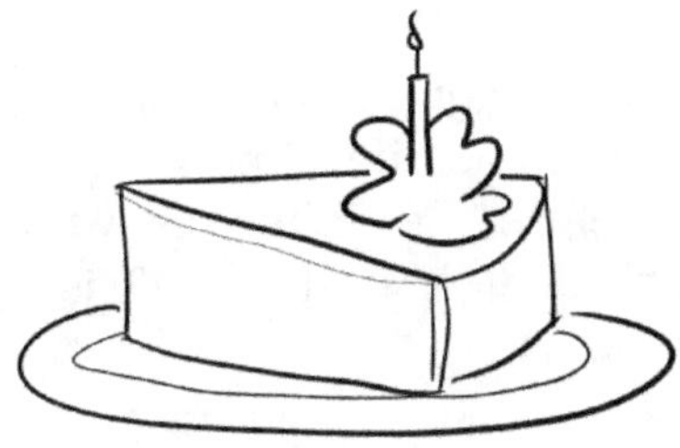

Change Just One Thing

Recently, I was asked to answer a few questions for a company that was looking to better understand people with diabetes. I expected a list of questions ranging from "What color meter do you prefer?" to "List all medications you are taking to treat your diabetes, and why."

Instead, the questions were more touchy-feely than I had anticipated. And a few of them were hard to answer. The one I struggled most with was "If you could change one thing about living with diabetes, what would it be?"

My first response was to shrug. "Everything? I'd change everything?"

Then I regrouped a bit. But still, an answer wasn't jumping into my head as easily as it had for the prior questions. Somehow, "What or who serves as your motivation or inspiration?" was much easier.

I'm only guessing, but I think if diabetes comes into your life when you are older, there's a distinct "before" and "after" to your life timeline. You remember when insulin injections or pumps or glucose meters weren't part of the equation. You know what it's like to drink juice purely for pleasure. You have a sense of what you're missing, of what's changed. I'd imagine that concept makes a diagnosis both easier and infinitely harder, on so many levels.

Diagnosed as a kid, I don't have many pre-diabetes memories at all. I'm not feel sorry for myself, but it's just a fact. I don't remember life without any of this medical stuff, and there is no "before." Just "after." Only the after part isn't this big dramatic change - it's just how life is.

So when asked what I'd change about living with diabetes, I don't have enough life without it to lay claim to a quality answer. I don't give a lot of thought to the meters or the pumps or all the physical trappings of diabetes. I don't mind because I don't know any differently.

But I wish I could lessen the emotional impact of diabetes on my life, and on the lives of the people I love.

I wish diabetes wasn't such a fickle mess, and that my mother could safely assume that I'll wake up just fine every morning. And that my husband wouldn't view the Dexcom as his safety net when he travels without me. And that I wouldn't have seeds of concern when I'm alone with my daughter. I wish this stupid disease didn't come with so much worry, and I really would love to change how that worry bleeds into the lives of my loved ones.

If I could tie diabetes to a balloon and let it soar out of my life, I totally would. If I could flush it down the toilet like a goldfish, I'd do that, too. I'd let a bear maul it. I'd allow my diabetes to stick a fork into a plugged-in toaster. And if I had the opportunity to shove it in a microwave like a Peep at Easter, I'd do it in a second. I'm not a fan of this disease, especially when it makes people worry.

I guess my first response was sort of right. "I'd change everything." ... only I'd add balloons, microwaves, and bears.

At Least It's Not ...

A recent community writing prompt included this: "If you could switch chronic diseases, which one would you choose to deal with instead of diabetes? And while we're considering other chronic conditions, do you think your participation in the DOC has affected how you treat friends and acquaintances with other medical conditions?"

This prompt makes me think of this: "Type 1 diabetes? At least it's not [insert other health condition here]."

I am not comfortable with this prompt. Mostly because it makes me feel lucky for how things are, and at the same time apprehensive about how they make shake out. And I can't reconcile those feelings; I can't bake them together into something I can swallow.

I feel lucky that, of all the chronic illnesses that I could be living with, I have type 1 diabetes. "Lucky" actually feels like a dirty word, the wrong word, and I wish there was a word that would better exemplify that it's not "luck," but thankfulness for treatment options, coupled with thankfulness that I was born and raised in a country where my educated, employed parents had access to not only the drug I needed to stay alive, but also the means to provide education that would help me make choices and decisions that contributed to improved health outcomes.

This thankfulness comes part and parcel with an appreciation for how invisible type 1 diabetes can be, and how I don't look, or feel, very sick on a day-to-day basis. I'm grateful that, even though my immune system has buckled in that one sense, I can survive. I feel lucky. This disease requires a lot of effort every day simply to hit stride with "normal," but most of the time, it's not something that keeps me from having a good day.

And exactly at the same time, every day is laced with an apprehension that I can't quite put my finger on. While low blood sugars are brief in duration, sometimes they are so intense and honestly scary that they leave me nervous for hours, or weeks, afterward. Sometimes the threat of a low is enough to kick apprehension into gear, like when I'm cramming extra glucose tabs into my exercise pack when I go for a run, picturing myself a few miles from home and wandering, disoriented and severely hypoglycemic. Before I go to bed at night, every single night, I check the IOB on my pump and the graph on my Dexcom and I try to calculate the probability of an overnight hypoglycemic event that might be easy and quick to treat, or that may be the moment that changes everything.

And while high blood sugars aren't comfortable while they play out, I am apprehensive about what that 150, 190, 250 ... 300 mg/dL does even during its brief visit. Even though my body appears to work and seems healthy, this disease makes my body unable to self-manage blood sugar levels, and sometimes the worry about what is happening to the actual cells of my body is enough to fill my mind with troubling thoughts about what may happen, despite my efforts. This apprehension now is without my dealing with marked complications, without other health conditions in play. And that makes me more apprehensive about how the future may unfold.

This disease is a mental bowl of marbles, some black with worry, some white with hope, but mostly filled with gray ones of varying shades, where worry and apprehension and hope and fear and joy and life mix together.

"At least it's not [insert other health condition here]."

But isn't that every health condition? Doesn't everyone who is living with a chronic health issue, or taking care of someone with one, deal with a very constant and unique thread of chaos and comfort, braided tightly?

I wouldn't want to switch with anyone. And I wouldn't want anyone to have to switch with me. I don't like anyone's body being compromised in any way. But at the same time, everyone who is managing a health "something" becomes part of my extended community.

Through diabetes, I hope I am learning about empathy, and hope, and not only other people's health conditions, but the human condition.

Full Body

The scar on my lower abdomen is close to healed, after six weeks of careful care. The incision is evidence of the arrival of my son, the same place my daughter escaped from. The skin above the incision is still swollen from months of pregnancy and oddly puckered due to surgery. It's not a flat, perfectly sculpted specimen of an abdomen.

But I try hard not to care. My kids were created here.

The marks on my fingertips move every few days as I use a lancet to draw blood every few hours. Sometimes the dots left behind look like I stuck my finger into a jar of ground pepper, other times they are light brown marks that appear to live deep beneath the surface of my skin.

But they represent moments when I needed to check my blood sugar and actually followed through on gathering that data. When I look at them, I see evidence of me taking good care of myself.

The scaly patches of skin on my outer thighs are itchy and refuse to respond to lovely lotions and dermatologist intervention. They are left behind by continuous glucose monitor sensors that I wear to keep tabs on my blood sugars throughout the day and night.

These skin issues are not comfortable or enviable, but the protection provided by streaming my glucose data helps me to sleep better.

My health is worth the inconvenient itch.

And, of course, there's the shifting of my body, shaped by time and illness and exercise and pregnancies. Baby weight. Aging, even when I don't remember to. My leg muscles are softer, but eager to be used again. My eyes have improved during this pregnancy, somehow. My blood pressure is carefully watched. My stomach is paunchier than it was 10 months ago.

I weigh myself to see what's happened over the last six weeks and try not to get too excited or sad at the result.

But the number on the scale doesn't define me. Neither does the number on my meter. Neither does my age.

... right?

I look at my body sometimes and feel a little embarrassed or ashamed because I don't physically conform to what magazine pages and commercials suggest I should look like. I'm not tall and willowy with shiny hair and slender arms. And I sort of, somewhat care about the size of the pants or the cut of the dress.

It's been harder than normal lately because I'm trying to recognize this new person in the mirror, the one who has carried two children and thirty years of chronic illness under her skin, never mind life's normal wear and tear.

I've lived with body image issues that haven't caused chaos but have given me pause from time to time. Diabetes has forced me to see my body through a specific lens, not always a rose-colored one. Sometimes diabetes makes me feel like I'm broken, unable to make insulin and struggling to create a child.

It's weird to look in the mirror and see someone who doesn't look sick but who has felt unwell physically many times, and who requires effort to stay emotionally well.

Other times, the diabetes lens makes me feel as if I have superpowers ... like, shouldn't I be dead because I don't make insulin? Every mile I've run or weight I've lifted stands in contrast to my unmotivated pancreas. How has my body managed to stop producing a life-sustaining hormone and yet I'm still here?

Can't I fly, too? And melt steel doors with my eyeball lasers?

I have to remind myself that there are marks and imperfections
on this body that I've fucking earned. There are a lot of scars.
Some visible, others harder to see, but all of them, earned or self-
imposed, have contributed to creating me. This body is
recovering from, responding to, reinventing itself in life, and
that's the image of my body I'm holding tight

The Gray Area

"Diabetes makes you a hero! You're pinch-hitting for a busted pancreas, and you're kicking ass! Nothing can stop you! Climb mountains, run marathons, compete, destroy threats, take no prisoners! The world is your oyster, and even with a busted pancreas, you remain the pearl!"

We see that. Or we hear ...

"Diabetes will eat you alive. Busted pancreas is only the beginning. Bring on the failing kidneys, the amputated limbs, the great-aunt Berthas who are the buried torsos you will become. Depression might join the party, too. And what about eating disorders? This shit will kill you and your efforts are a nice try, but get ready for the ground."

Intense messages. Both sentiments have their truths. Diabetes can be a blip on your badass radar and it can also kill you. It's both of those things. It's all of these things. I don't have my head in the sand about what's possible, on either side of the spectrum.

I live entirely in the gray area, in the middle.

I am not recently diagnosed. Diagnosed as a kid, I have 31 years of lived experience with type 1 diabetes. My health is good but it remains a work in progress (still working on shedding some of this baby weight, also working on an A1C reboot, need to continue to work on managing anxiety, and am living with diabetes-related eye complications).

I'm not climbing any mountains but I can do a few miles on the treadmill and I successfully created two human beings, so I'm feeling good about that.

Aspirational? Not really. You won't find carefully curated diabetes on my social media feeds because my diabetes is not always nice to look at. Defeated? Not even a little bit. I don't want emails telling me that diabetes will be my cause of death because that is not a source of motivation for me. I'm in somewhat of a gray area, the middle ground, rejecting fear and embracing hope.

I still have a lot of hope. A lot. I think good things are coming for people with diabetes, delivered by diabetes devices and drug development and advocacy efforts and stories that are shared by our community. And what makes viewing my good health as a work in progress instead of an impossible dream is that hope. I am aware of the terrible things that diabetes can to do a person, and to a family, and my hope doesn't minimize those things.

Instead, my hope serves as fuel in time when the news cycle is beyond bleak. Hope is what makes me check my blood sugar and change out my insulin pump infusion set. It's what makes me cook up a healthy meal. It's what prompts me to go to the gym. It's what makes me want to share my diabetes story and hear stories from others. Hope is both a safety net and a shield against the fear.

Hope makes my efforts feel like they're in pursuit of an outcome worth fighting for. With no cure currently on deck for diabetes, my daily determination to make my health a priority is rooted in that hope.

Because the world is your oyster, and even with a busted pancreas, you remain the pearl.

Voicemail for my Pancreas

"Hey, you. This is awkward. Voicemail. I hate voicemail. But I haven't heard from you in a while ... almost like 30 years now, actually.

How the hell have you been? It's been busy over here – a lot has happened since second grade. I finished elementary school. I learned how to tap dance but the whole soccer thing never really worked out. Graduated high school, graduated college ... I got married! I have a kid – she's almost six. I have another one on the way.

There's been a lot. A lot has happened.

I know you're in there. Mostly because the other stuff you're supposed to be doing, with all the enzymes and all that stuff, is still happening so I know you're alive. Just not doing the insulin thing.

But that's cool. I used to be angry about it, but I'm kind of over it. Maybe not over it, but I'm apathetic. Like I don't care that you aren't answering my calls these days – I don't really want to talk-talk to you, but sometimes I would just like to say hi, punch you in your non-face face, and then move on.

But that's not an option. All I can do is keep going. Keep checking blood sugars and taking insulin and doing the diabetes thing. Working. Growing this new kid as best I can and taking care of my daughter, too. Doing the life thing. Holding up my end of that bargain, at least.

I'm kind of glad you didn't answer. I don't even know if you'll listen to this, and I don't really care if you do. That apathy thing; It felt good to say hi. And that I don't mind you being gone. I miss you – I'm fucking frustrated without you sometimes – but I don't need you.

Okay, I feel better. Sorry for leaving this on your voicemail. See you around."

Click.

"Hey again. Sorry – one last thing. I'm done saving all your fucking mail, by the way. Who gets that many catalogs? And you owe the endocrinologist like a million dollars. Might want to follow up on some of those bills. Bye."

Healthcare
Experiences

Healthcare Experiences

A few years ago, I started seeing a new endocrinologist and we clicked pretty well. I told a colleague that I felt like this endo could also be a quasi-friend.

"A friend-o," I said, rolling the thought around in my mind.

That's the best-case scenario for an endo, right? Someone who you can work well with? Someone you trust? A friendocrinolgist!

My visits with clinicians are more than just doctor appointments to me. They are pockets of time where I partner with healthcare specialists to work on this lifelong science experiment of life with diabetes. Doctor appointments can be humbling, and awkward, and stressful, but they're in pursuit of maintaining good health, so follow-through and good communication are key.

... but sometimes the healthcare system itself can make the whole arrangement complicated. It's expensive. It's reactive. It's a hot mess. Finding the right doctor/patient partnership can be challenging with you're trying to navigate the nuances and frustrations of industrialized healthcare.

Being a patient can be hard work. And making sense of the healthcare system is also hard. These stories touch upon what it's like to be a patient with chronic illness, about the relationship with our trusted clinical advisors, and how mutual respect goes a long way.

Lies

I used to lie to my pediatric endocrinologist. I am not proud of this.

She'd sit at her desk and look through the logbook with all my blood sugars mapped out (this was back in the day when my mom and I collaborated on logging my blood sugars, which meant that they were often accounted for), sometimes with a furrowed brow.

"There are a lot of higher numbers in the morning, after breakfast. Do you think we need to look at that morning insulin-to-carb ratio? Maybe that needs some tweaking, to help with these post-breakfast numbers."

There was a good, full year (or two) when I was a teenager and I would meet with my pediatric endocrinologist, having these strong, intelligent conversations about blood sugars and ratios and numbers. She and I would crunch numbers and make changes, all in pursuit of lowering my A1C (which, as a teenager, swung wildly). I talked the talk. I sounded like a gave a shit.

But in reality, I was lying to my excellent doctor. I was wasting her time.

I would show up for my appointments in full-swing teenage diabetes rebellion, knowing exactly why my post-breakfast numbers were such shit but still not able to admit to my endocrinologist that the reason my blood sugars were high after breakfast was because I was too lazy/disinterested/foolish teenager to properly count my carbs. I was a very privileged teenager in that I had access to excellent diabetes care at the Joslin Clinic, a stash of insulin and glucose meter test strips in my bathroom closet at home, and a family that was both interested in and dedicated to my health and well-being.

So why the hell was I lying to my endo? Why was I fifteen years old, talking with my kind endocrinologist about numbers that looked dodgy on paper but weren't entirely riddles wrapped in mysteries – these numbers were the product of actively distancing myself from the responsibility of diabetes self-care. The answer was clear – the insulin-to-carb ratios were probably fine and I was just SWAG-bolusing – so why wasn't I fessing up and saving my endo the effort of trying to find "a solution?"

Yesterday, I was in Minneapolis, Minnesota giving a keynote presentation at the Annual ICSI Colloquium on Health Care Transformation and part of my talk was about how – and why – patients sometimes lie to their doctors. Like when I lied to my peds endocrinologist about my post-breakfast blood sugars, or how I've also lied about how much regular exercise I was getting throughout the course of a week. ("Exercising every day? Yes! With bells on! Um ... weighted bells!")

These lies aren't told to in efforts to be malicious, but more because it's hard to admit failure, especially to people I respect. It's also hard to admit it to myself. I liked my pediatric endocrinologist very, very much and I didn't want her to think my lack of diabetes follow-through, at times, was because I was a bad person. It was hard to explain to her how much I wanted her to like working with me, and to be proud of me, as part of our patient-HCP relationship. It was hard to explain why I ignored the daily duties of diabetes sometimes, even though I didn't want to ignore them. It just didn't make sense. A lot of the time, I didn't want her to think I was a jerk, like I was wasting her time or something (even though the lies did waste her time – it was a vicious cycle).

"The reason it's easier to be honest with my endocrinologist now is because she views my pancreas as non-compliant, not me." I told the ICSI group. "As a patient, I didn't want to disappoint my doctor. It took a long time to realize that the lies didn't help improve my health."

Embracing honesty with my current endo has been difficult, but necessary. I'm able to tell her when I'm going through diabetes burnout, or when I'm skimping on different aspects of my self-care. It took a long time to make me feel as though honesty was the best policy because it actually enabled my doctor and I to address the things I needed help with, instead of pretending that everything was fine.

I wish I had been as forthcoming with my pediatric endo as I am with my adult endo, but it's still hard, even now, to look her in the eye and admit the stupid mistakes I make. Maybe that's part of the "growing up with diabetes" education curve, learning that I can't aim to fix what I won't acknowledge.

I have a feeling that learning curve goes on forever.

Just a Job

"I'm just a medical assistant, so my job isn't as important," she said as she took my blood pressure and entered the data into my digital file.

"Seriously? How can you say that? You probably have more face-to-face time with patients than the doctors do. You set the tone for the appointment. What you do matters." I paused. "Take my blood pressure again," I laughed. "It probably just went up."

She smiled. "I guess it is important. But not as important as the doctor."

It's strange how people think their interactions don't matter, don't have an influence on the patient experience.

When the receptionist checks me in for my appointment, she contributes to the tone of my appointment. Even if she is asking me for my insurance information for the tenth time, or informing me of an outstanding balance on my account, or telling me that the doctor is running late today, the way she delivers that information colors the experience.

When the phlebotomist is steady-handed and double-checks the information on the blood vial label against my file, their attention to detail and dedication to comfort colors the experience.

When the medical assistant makes eye contact, engages the patient, and acknowledges that the data they are collecting is from a human being, not a lab rat, they color the experience.

When the clinician is on time and the appointment is not an exercise in redundancy and checked boxes on an electronic medical record but instead a discussion between a patient and a provider that influences positive health outcomes, that interaction colors the experience.

And when I'm on time, and I have the necessary and requested data from my diabetes devices, when I have my list of questions and concerns, when I pay my bill or file my claim, and when I'm respectful of everyone's time and expertise, I color the experience.

There is no "just a ..." when it comes to the healthcare experience. Even when it's not medically coded as a "shared medical appointment," the appointment is still shared between the patient and everyone their interact with. Everyone involved makes or breaks those moments for the patient and the healthcare team alike, with each person playing a crucial role in keeping the process effective, efficient, and evolving.

Time-Consuming

"Thank you for calling [insert every company name I had to call yesterday here]. Please listen carefully, as our telephone options have changed."

"Please press one to continue in English, para español, marque dos."

"Press three if you are a patient, press four if you are a provider, press five if you are a member of the media, press six to return to the main menu, press one if you noticed that we skipped right to three and didn't mention two."

"Enter your twelve digit prescription number."

"Enter your date of birth."

"I'm sorry – your date of birth is not valid. Please re-enter your date of birth starting with a two digit month, two digit date, and four digit year."

"Enter your six digit group number, followed by the date of birth of the primary policy holder."

"What is your shipping address?"

"I'm sorry – I didn't understand that. Can you please confirm your shipping address?"

"Your shipment will be to you in seven to ten business days. One of your orders requires special packaging and will arrive on your doorstep wrapped in pillows of ice with penguins stamped on the side and your neighbors might think you have ice cream delivered every three months in bulk but you and I both know it's just insulin – wink, wink."

"Your confirmation number will be given to you at the end of this call. Please be sure to write that confirmation number down."

"If you'd like to enroll in our automatic refill program, please listen to the following message. If you don't want to enroll in our automatic refill program, please listen to this message because you can't hang up until you hear the confirmation number."

"Please hold while we process your request. Do not disconnect before hearing your confirmation number."

"Your confirmation number is the sum of 5+4-(323 x 423)/9. Would you like me to repeat your confirmation number?"

"Press three to speak with a customer service representative."

"Are you sure? Press three again, twice and really fast, to speak with a customer service representative."

"Please hold while we transfer your call."

"Thank you for continuing to hold. Please continue to hold."

"Thank you for holding. We heard you pee; you weren't on mute. Thank you for washing your hands. Please continue to hold."

"Hoooooooooooooold."

"Still hold."

...

...

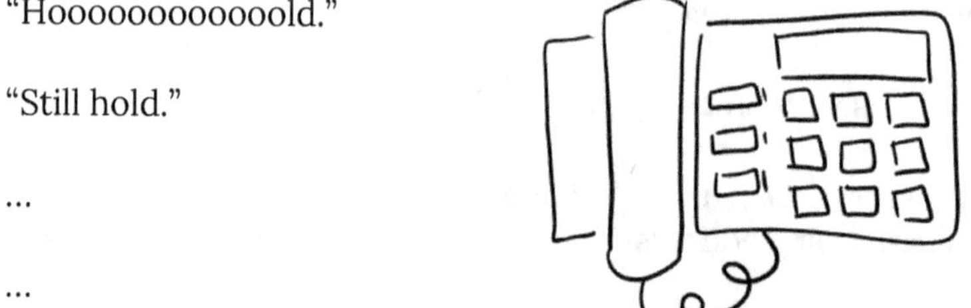

"Thank you for calling. Please listen carefully, as our telephone options have changed."

Trapped by Shipments and Timeouts

Day-to-diabetes requires a lot of focus on timing; what time did I take my insulin, what time did I eat, what time will I exercise, what time will I be in a meeting, what time am I planning to go to bed, what time will my insulin and my food seemingly serendipitously meet somewhere in my body, mapping out into my bloodstream ... the list of things to be timed is on-going.

Pinch-hitting for a misfiring pancreas is the embodiment of the White Rabbit.

The healthcare/medical device system adds a few new yards to this rabbit hole I'm tumbling down. This past week, I had a G6 sensor fall off after only four days of wear, with only one sensor in house. I had to wait five days until I could reorder, opening a weird timing window.

Will I receive new sensors before the 10 days are up on this current one? Nope, because there's a backorder at Dexcom.

Should I open the last G5 transmitter and use my last box and a half of G5 sensors? Mmmm, unsure because that would start the 90-day timer on that transmitter and then I'd be running out the clock on the last 3 weeks of my G6 transmitter and THIS SHIT COSTS $$$ and I value what I earn and what I spend on diabetes care and do not want to waste a moment of use with these pricey devices.

I was away for the last few days and while I was gone, the replacement sensor for the G6 sensor that wept off my skin arrived. Ten more days of wear, starting tomorrow morning, still within the window of using my current transmitter.

But the clock continues to tick on to the next ordering deadline, the next scheduled payment, the next copay, the next quarterly insurance debit, the next open enrollment, the next held breath to make sure necessities are covered, the next time that diabetes makes me think more about my wallet than my pancreas.

How to Improve my Healthcare Experience

What would improve the healthcare experience for me, as a patient with multiple health conditions? I'm glad you asked. (You did actually ask, right?) A few things would help move things forward. Here's a thought-purging because I happened to have coffee:

Billing processes that make sense. For example, I received a refund for mail order pharmacy overpayment in the same week I received a collection notice for the same account. I had overpaid because their receivables system wasn't as fast as their billing system, which flagged my account for collections when in fact I was ahead of the game. If the billing system was synced properly with the accounts receivable system, they would have known I was in the black, not in the red.

But thanks for sending all those letters telling me I wouldn't receive any more insulin shipments unless I paid the (not due) balance. (Also, get paid for things that make sense. A test to diagnose me with type 1 diabetes twenty-nine years after my type 1 diabetes diagnosis is ridiculous, but required by my insurance company. What a waste of resources. Spoiler alert: I have type 1 diabetes.)

Everyone be on time. Simple, right? If my appointment is at 10 am, I show up no later than 9.45 am, usually 9.30 am. I'm afraid of being late. But the HCP showing up at 10:15, 10:30 ... 11 am is fine because their schedule takes precedence over mine? I understand being late from time to time, but a 10 am appointment should not linger well into lunch time. I like lunch too much to miss it.

Make getting paid easier. My doctors should be paid for what they do. If they review my CGM data, there should be a billing code that pays them for that review. If they (by the grace of some fancy god) are able to email me, they should be paid for sending that email. Their medical expertise is hard-earned and should be properly appreciated.

To that same end, my insurance company should pay out (incentivize!) proactive care instead of reacting to chaos. My parents should not have had to battle for more than three test strips per day for me when I was a kid. Checking my blood sugar should be fully covered, as it's an investment in keeping me healthy. Pay to keep my body whole; don't start paying only once it falls apart.

Don't let money drive every decision. Twice in the last three months, I've had to make appointments with new care providers and the very, very first question out of the receptionist's mouth is, "What insurance do you have?" This is immediately after, "Hello?" I would guess that this is in effort to streamline the phone tree (and triage) process, but you don't even know why I'm calling. And you have no idea what I can and cannot pay for. Asking if you'll be paid before asking if I'm okay puts financial needs in the driver's seat ... yet another driver, with the patient tied up in the trunk.

Treat me where I am. If I come into my GP's office with an issue that applies to their primary care practice but they consider it a diabetes-related issue and they refer me back to my endo in order to receive care, that's crap. Treat the patient where they are. Ask about and then make the mental health referral in my endo's office, please.

Don't turn me away if I come to my PCP with a diabetes need. Sometimes it's difficult to get time off to go to the appointment, and having the issue not even addressed because it's deemed out of scope makes it that much harder for me, as a patient, to coordinate care.

Integrate all the things. My A1C should be sent by my endo to my primary care doctor's office. My pregnancy file should be sent from the high-risk maternal fetal medicine office that delivered Birdy to my "regular" OB/GYN here in Rhode Island. (Why am I still tracking that information down, almost six years later?) My dental records should be on file at my PCP's office. Any visit with a mental health professional should be documented and sent to my PCP and my endo.

I'm not asking my medical teams to start a softball team, but it would be good if my information flowed in a predictable and useful way. Instead, I have this weird folding file of information and lab work and notes in my phone, creating a patchwork quilt of my medical information that's a little threadbare. It would be great if EMRs (or EHRs or EMFs) actually worked for me, and for my medical team. Otherwise, they become another tool that keeps my medical team from making eye contact with me and I'm still dragging around that folding file.

Life with chronic illness has taught me that the medical system is broken. This isn't a hard and fast fact, but anecdotal experiences often harden into truth. And that truth is what my life with diabetes is really like.

A Cleaning

"Your appointment is at ... at 2 pm."

"Yes."

"It's 1.30 pm. You're a little bit early." The receptionist looked up at me. "No one is ever early."

"I was afraid that if I didn't come early, I would have found a reason to skip the appointment entirely. I'm a little nervous about dental stuff," I admitted, trying to stand taller and look more like a grown-up instead of like a kid whose mother had to drop her off at the door. (For the record, I drove there myself.)

The receptionist outright laughed. "Oh, a nervous one! That's okay. We have a lot of magazines. And you can watch the stories on TV while you wait for the hygienist."

Anyone who refers to daytime soap operas as "the stories" puts me right at ease. I sat in the waiting room and played Candy Crush (fake candy doesn't count against my teeth, right?) while waiting for the dentist.

Back in January, after an unfortunate and wimpy two-year dental hiatus, I found my way back into the dentist's chair as a result of social media peer pressure. I've written about my aversion to dental work in the past, my reluctance rooted in the fact that my overly-sensitive teeth make for a very uncomfortable experience. But, despite a long gap between appointments, I had a good experience a few months ago, which was encouraging enough to make me schedule, and keep, a follow up appointment.

An empowered patient doesn't always rabble-rouse and shout from rooftops about patient rights and experiences. Sometimes being an empowered patient is simply speaking up on your own behalf. Part of what has made going to the dentist a better experience for me is that I'm not afraid to tell the dentist what I'm hoping to get out of the appointment.

(Even though my fear comes out via stream of consciousness, when I'm halfway sitting in the chair and blurting out, "I don't meant to sound neurotic but I sort of am when it comes to dental work because I have really, really sensitive teeth and I had a few dentists in the past do some work on my teeth that didn't go very well, so now every dental appointment makes me nervous and if that pointy sharp mental thing comes too close to my gum line I will probably launch right up through the really nice skylights you guys have – and those are really expensive to fix, right? Skylights?")

And the other part of what makes these appointments a better experience is that my dentist, and their team, really listens and takes patient comfort into account.

"It doesn't cost us anything extra to take the time to listen and make your appointment something you're willing to do again," the hygienist said. "If anything, it's an investment in our future, because if you continue to come back, you become part of our reliable client base, and that's a good thing for us, as a business."

Being on top of my health means making sure I follow through on things like dentist appointments. Proactive care for my health makes a difference in long term outcomes, but I need to do my part by showing up.

Having a dentist that I can be honest with ("I'm scared of you ... no offense meant?") makes us work together to find ways to make the appointment more comfortable – numbing cream on my gums during the cleaning, safely administering extra Novocain as needed during procedures – which, in turn, makes me show up at the next appointment. Having a dentist is useless if I'm not going to see them.

"Everything looks good. Do you want to schedule your follow-up appointment today, or call in a few weeks?"

"I'll do it today ..."

"To make sure that you actually schedule it," the dentist finished for me.

"Right. Otherwise, I'll never come back."

"And we can't have that," the dentist said, ruefully. "Because then I'd never know how much it costs to fix a skylight."

Being a Rotten Patient

Yesterday, I was a rotten patient.

At this point in my previous pregnancy, I had already been in hospital on bedrest for two weeks, so this whole rolling around on the "outside" while a few days shy of 37 weeks pregnant is new to me. The emotions I felt on bedrest were really volatile and I cried a lot and HEY that same shit keeps happening even though I'm not on bedrest currently. Which means that my third trimester experiences are consistent, at least emotionally.

Which sets the stage for yesterday. I had an appointment at the maternal fetal medicine offices and then at my endocrinologist, both up in Boston. Usually, the ride takes me about an hour and 45 minutes, but I give myself 2 hours and 15 minutes every time, to anticipate traffic. Yesterday, the ride took two and a half hours because of wicked traffic on Brookline Avenue, which made me late for my scheduled ultrasound.

I do not like to be late. And yesterday, being late made me all emotional. My car crawled up Brookline Avenue while I imagined having to reschedule my appointment for the following day, making the stupid drive all over again. By the time I pulled into the parking garage, I had six minutes to find the right hospital wing and check in for my appointment.

Which, of course, I did not do efficiently. Late pregnancy hormones and emotions have my brain mostly scrambled, so I ended up in the wrong wing of the clinic, nowhere near where I was supposed to be.

My blood sugar started to tumble at this point, bringing emotions even more to the surface while I left a trail of glucose tab dust along the hallways of Beth Israel. Add that to the fact that I was late and mildly lost in the myriad of signs and corridors and I lost my cool.

Man, I felt stupid. I was crying while waddling through the hospital, asking random people how to get to the proper hospital wing. Their directions weren't making sense to my slightly hypoglycemic head. I could not pull myself together, awash with frustration and embarrassment and unable to control the emotional maelstrom swirling around me.

I was unjustifiably angry that the best care for myself and my kid included a four-hour road trip for every doctor's visit. I was so tired from the low blood sugars that kept me up from 3 – 5 am and were the most symptomatic I've had in ages. I was angry that I couldn't guarantee safety for my child as a result of my own health garbage. I was afraid that the stress of the moment was kicking my blood pressure into dangerous ranges. I was a frightful mess and it wasn't anyone's fault but mine but holy moly, I was blowing up balloons by the dozen for this ridiculous pity party I was throwing for myself.

By the time I arrived at the right place, I was 15 minutes late and trembling. And angry. When the nurses were waiting outside of the bathroom to grab me for my appointment, I snapped at them. When they took my blood pressure while I was crying (could NOT stop for some reason), I knew the result would be elevated and would trigger a whole catalog of panicked responses from my healthcare team. Of course it was high, and of course I snapped at them again. Not their fault that I was late and my BP was high, yet they were the unfortunate recipients of my rage.

When the nurse I've been working with and a new doctor came in to discuss the results of my ultrasound (baby is fine) and my blood pressure (elevated for reasons I knew but they couldn't pretend it couldn't be a symptom of preeclampsia), I was still ranting and snappy I could not calm down and I felt terrible – TERRIBLE – that I was lashing out at a medical team whose purpose was to protect my health and the health of my baby.

But I still couldn't get my shit together and acknowledge that for more than five minutes.

I was a rotten patient, all frustrated and angry. (The ultrasound technician told me it was okay and that they see a lot of emotions during appointments, and I felt myself simultaneously apologize and then get all upset again. No control.) I snapped at healthcare professionals who were not to blame for my terrible mood. I could not control my emotional responses to their reasonable requests. I'm embarrassed at how I acted.

I hate admitting all of this.

The appointment circuit was finished later that afternoon, after everyone had reached the conclusion that I was able to go home until the next appointment (later this week) and reassess then. I apologized to the people I had acted bananas towards and drove home, hoping to be more emotionally stable the next time.

I need to see this pregnancy through safely, but the last nine months have really opened my eyes to what I need to receive, as a patient, and just as importantly, what I need to bring to the table, as a patient. Sometimes I can't effectively perform as a full-time pregnant person, or a full-time person with diabetes (and clearly I'm struggling with doing both of those things at the moment), and I need to own that part of my healthcare experience.

Or at least stop crying in the stupid elevators, making everyone on there with me think I'm about to give birth in front of them.

Share and Don't Share

"I'm sorry," "thank you," and "please" are the thematic statements of every endocrinologist appointment I have.

"Thank you." You're great. You really are. I've been a patient of yours for years now and your patience for your patients knows no bounds. You're also smart, as you've been dealing with adults with type 1 for a long time, and you rarely view my diabetes as something that happens outside of the context of all the other stuff in my life. "You don't live in a vacuum," and I always laugh in my head because I picture Henry the Vacuum (look him up), and it's a hard mental image to shake.

You don't give me the stink eye when I tell you I don't have weeks' worth of logbooks available, but you do make me own the fact that you need at least two weeks of certain numbers (fasting, before meals, before bed) to make assessments of my blood sugar needs. Accountability helps, and I at least know what the bare minimum data points that you need are. Because of your prowess when it comes to type 1 diabetes and pregnancy (and all of the assorted fun-and-games that can crop up in tandem), I was confident in trusting you to help bring my dream of motherhood to a healthy fruition.

"I'm sorry." Even though I cry in your office almost every time, you don't make me feel creepy about it. I don't know what it is - pent up anxiety? emotions that I keep bottled becoming uncorked when your office door shuts? - but it's a knee-jerk response. My emotional response to diabetes seems to rear its head when we're talking about the basic mechanics, because I think I'm frustrated at the fact that being "compliant" doesn't always lead to awesome lab work results. Or peace. Or more sleep. Or any guaranteed awesome.

And I'm also sorry for being a sometimes-scatterbrained patient. I know the point of my being there is to review numbers, and make adjustments to medications, etc. and I do feel horrible when I don't come armed with all the information you need to help me make sense of diabetes. However, our relationship is a two-way one, and even though we have a good repertoire, there are things we can work on.

"Please." Please don't think that my scattered records equal out to apathy about day-to-day diabetes management. (I test my blood sugar, but I don't always log it. And I take my insulin, even though I'm not always plotting the doses on a spreadsheet.) Please find a way for your office - the insurance company? - to reimburse you for reviewing CGM data. Please don't leave me waiting in your office for over an hour, finally starting a 10 am appointment at 11:30 am - I'm supposed to be 15 minutes early, but it's okay if you're 90 minutes late? Please ask your office staff to respect the fact that I may not know all the details of what is and isn't covered by my insurance, and please encourage them to treat me respectfully when I call to make appointments/ask a question. Please don't judge me for changing my lancet every *mumble mumble*.

Doctor/patient relationships are just that: relationships. I think ours is good. I am confident I am getting good care from you, and I hope you feel that I'm a patient worth dedicating your time to. Type 1 diabetes takes a fair amount of work to manage, and I'm thankful to have you on my team.

Things You Eat and Things that Beep

Things You Eat and Things That Beep

In my experiences, diabetes gave food a lot of emotional assignments. Food can be the villain, the hero, the antihero, the distributor of desire and guilt. I ate in secret when I was growing up. I had a lot of guilt about food choices and some self-consciousness about body perceptions. I was encouraged to only eat "healthy foods" unless my blood sugar was tanking, and then I was told to grab the nearest bag of Skittles. The emotional range attached to a banana is truly astounding.

Diabetes puts a strange shine on what we eat, and I often explore that through writing.

(I struggled to break these essays into two different sections, mostly because I didn't have enough of either type to justify separate sections. Hence the mash-up of food-related essays and diabetes technology. Hence the weird section title. Hence this next bit about technology and its beeping boopness.)

I've also included pieces on diabetes technology into this section because there's emotions assigned to those inanimate objects, too. My diabetes wearable technology has been a source of both pride and struggle for me over the years, their intrusion making diabetes management more streamlined while making getting dressed kind of complicated. Wearable diabetes technology bits were my first visible symptom of diabetes, and adjusting to that change took time.

Ready to get emotionally weird about snacks and tech? Let's do it.

Crabs

Crabs are something that people with diabetes are constantly grappling with. Are crabs good for us? Should we be avoiding crabs at all costs? If we have too many crabs in our diet, will our A1c go up? What's the official recommendation for diabetics as it pertains to crabs? Has anyone ever really tamed the wild crabs? Is anyone eating crabs, right now, as they read this?

(Note: Spellcheck is my nemesis right now. It always, always wants to change "carbs" to "crabs." Spellcheck also likes changing "bolusing" to "blousing," as if wearing a puffy shirt is a verb. For the record, I have nothing against crabs. Crabs are fine. And, in my opinion, carbs are fine, too. Spellcheck is a bit of a bitch, though.)

I've been told, time and time again, that carbs are evil. That if I maintain a diet that's reasonably low-carb, my diabetes will thank me for it. But I don't think that carbohydrates are the enemy. In fact, they're my best molecular friend when my blood sugar is hanging out in the trenches.

But.

I did notice, as I was gearing up for my wedding and working out more than usual, that my very low carb diet and my consistent exercise regimen made for minimal spikes in my blood sugar. It wasn't a perfect system, but subbing in vegetables for mashed potatoes at dinner time made for a post-prandial under 200 mg/dl, which (pre-BSparl), was a solid goal for me.

Granted, I didn't avoid carbs all the time, but I actively avoided high carb diet choices because I knew both my weight and my A1c would pay the price somehow.

And now, post-baby, I'm trying to go back to that lower carb lifestyle, because that helped keep me at a weight I was more comfortable with. (Not that I'm actively avoiding carbs now, thanks to the epic breastfeeding lows that crop up every few hours, so I'm giving myself a big ol' bell curve on getting back into a shape I like most.)

For me, part of the carbohydrate conundrum is user error. Pre-Bsparl, I could be a lazy boluser. I never bolused well in advance of a meal, and my post-prandials (and my overall A1C) definitely paid the price on repeat. It seems that I need to get my insulin pushed through my system at least 25 minutes before I sit down to eat, not five minutes before. I learned this lesson (23 years too late, eh?) while I planning for baby, and during the course of the pregnancy, it was definitely the case. Bolusing well before the meal worked better for me.

To each diabetic their own when it comes to carbohydrate intake. Some people are able to manage high piles of carbs without the messy spikes. Other people, like me, might be clumsy with their insulin. Or sometimes the decision not to carb has nothing to do with diabetes (as in my case, and in the case of my husband) - we go lower carb for weight management reasons. But there's no set magical diabetes diet that cures all that ails you.

Eating carbs, or not eating carbs, is a personal decision that each individual diabetic needs to figure out for themselves.

Froast

When I'm getting ready to go to the gym at night, I change up into my workout clothes and then test my blood sugar. For a cardio workout, I like to at least start in the 160 - 180 mg/dl range, but sometimes my numbers are lower than that at 6 pm.

Chris makes his protein shake and we talk about stuff that happened that day.

"So I was talking with [CoWorker] about this thing at work and ..." I lick the blood off my finger and see a result of 98 mg/dl. I walk over to the freezer and open up the bag of whole wheat bread, grabbing a slice. Still talking, though.

"... it could really help bolster community so we were thinking about making that our next project. What do you think?" I bite into cold, almost completely frozen slice of bread, the chill making it easy to swallow. Chew, chew, chew - all set.

"Good idea. Also, you'll be good to go in a few minutes?"

"Yeah. Having some froast and I'm good to go."

Froast. Frozen toast. I eat this all the time and only now am I realizing how (perhaps) slightly unusual it is. Doesn't everyone get their carbohydrate fix by chomping into a frozen slice of whole wheat bread, sans butter or jam or any kind of condiment?

Chris thinks this is the oddest thing, but I do it all the time and barely think anything of it anymore.

"Wouldn't it be fread? Like frozen bread?"

We have this discussion more often than two creative people with social skills should.

"No, because it's frozen. That's what makes it firm. So it's like toast, only not crispy from heat. More solid from cold."

Not "fread." Not "broast." Not "brozen." FROAST. It's a frigging weirdo staple in my diet.

Froast is a way for me to grab some carbs and keep my blood sugar holding a bit steadier instead of downing fast-acting slugs of juice and empty calories. I hate the idea of drinking my calories and would much rather have a good old-fashioned slice of froast. At least it's something of substance.

Froasty goodness!

Grocery Wars

The wheels on the grocery cart clatter against the store's tile floor as my Internal Motivational Speaker and My Stomach wage war inside my head.

Internal Motivational Speaker: Oh Kerri, don't those organic cucumbers look delicious! You can slice them up and eat them as a snack in the morning. Grab two of those.

My hands extend out and grab two cucumbers.

Stomach: Seriously, dude, if you don't get me something to eat I am going to make that noise you hate. You know the one.

Internal Motivational Speaker: And raspberries! They are filled with flavonoids. Get those, too.

The raspberries make their way into my cart. I shuffle through the grocery store on autopilot.

Internal Motivational Speaker: Yes, yes. Baby spinach. Some sliced turkey and cheese for sandwiches for lunch. Good idea. Baby carrots ...

Stomach: Baby spinach, baby carrots. You eat babies. Heh heh. FEED ME. I'm running out of patience.

I turn right and make my way down the granola bar and cereal aisle.

Internal Motivational Speaker: You liked those organic granola bars we bought last week. Grab another box of those. Keep walking past that cereal, too high in carbs for you. You know if makes you spike. How about some banana bread oatmeal? That worked out nicely.

The area just below my belly button lets loose with a low growl, like I'm hiding a ravenous bear underneath my workout shirt.

Stomach: See? Told you. You can't go to the gym and then come straight here without feeding me. I've let the bear loose now. That guy over there just looked at you because it sounds like you are about to throw up. Ha ha ha. Because you eat babies.

Internal Motivational Speaker: Stomach, stop being so crude! We'll be home soon. Just be patient.

Stomach: I am being patient. You don't know what I've been through, lady. She did abs tonight. Do you know what that means? She spent way too much time crunching and now I'm all tense. Hey Kerri, grab those frosted mini-wheats. I've earned them.

Internal Motivational Speaker: No, no! Frosting on the outside means high blood sugars on the inside, you moron!

Stomach: They say whole grain. Do you see that, Kerri? Whole. Grain. Grab 'em.

Whispering "Whole grains are in these," to myself, I add the mini-wheats to my cart.

Internal Motivational Speaker: I can't believe this! You just went to the gym and now you're adding frosted mini-wheats to the cart? I mean really, Kerri, you need to get your priorities straight. Now come on and put them back.

Stomach: Kerri, you have your priorities in fine order. You are eating well and exercising and torturing the hell out of me. Add those mini-wheats to your rabbit food carriage and let's get on with this. I need a snack.

The bear growls again.

Stomach: Rocco's getting upset. Better move on.

I move the mini-wheats underneath the bags of fresh vegetables. My Internal Motivational Speaker sighs deeply.

Internal Motivational Speaker: I can still see them, you know.

Stomach: Oh would you just shut up?

Internal Motivational Speaker: I will not. And another thing …

I hear the sound of a heavy chain snapping and the ravenous roar of a hungry bear.

Stomach: Sick 'em, Rocco!

Internal Motivational Speaker: Noooo!! Oh God, I can feel his breath on my motivational neck! Help!

Her voice trails off. The mini-wheats stay in the cart.

Rocco Returns

I should have packed more food. What was I thinking, bringing lunch only? Oh man, am I hungry.

Internal Motivational Speaker: Kerri, Kerri. You have a delicious spread of portabella chicken and spinach for lunch, complete with a drizzled bit of balsamic dressing. Can't you just have your lunch early?

Stomach: Give it up, Speaker. It's snack time. Snack time never includes healthy. Snack time is ravenous. Kerri, go downstairs and get a peppermint patty from the diner.

But I don't even like peppermint patties. I want a Nutrigrain bar.

Stomach: I don't care if you like it or not. It's almost ten-thirty. You've given me nothing but coffee. Rocco doesn't like coffee, Kerri.

Growling from the pits of my stomach. The chain rattles and I can hear him breathing heavily, scraping his paws along the floor.

Internal Motivational Speaker: (*panicked squeal*) Oh, hi Rocco! I see you have a new chain and collar. That's a lovely new chain. (*nervous laugh*) Have you done something different with your fur?

Rocco growls and leans against his chain, the links straining against one another.

Stomach: Easy there, Roc. It's cool, buddy. Kerri is going to go downstairs and grab you a Nutrigrain bar. You like those, don'tcha?

Rocco puffs out his bear breath and plunks down on his haunches, waiting. My stomach lurches a bit. I need something to eat. I get up from my desk chair and grab a dollar from my wallet. Rocco starts to purr, after a fashion.

Internal Motivational Speaker: Oh no. No, no Miss Kerri. Nutrigrain bars have high fructose corn syrup in them. Not to mention almost 25 grams of carbohydrates. You have that package of almonds in your drawer. Why not snack on those? Do you really need a high-carb indulgence right now? I mean ...

Stomach: Lady, do you ever take a breath? Let the girl have her Nutrigrain bar. It's not like she's going to have a side of soft-serve ice cream with it.

Internal Motivational Speaker: I am sick and tired of you bossing me around! I don't care that you have your fancy pepsinogen and that Pyloric sphincter. *(her voice crescendos to a vehement peak)* You aren't the boss of me. I have every right to my opinions!

Stomach: All you do is nag! Eat this, don't eat that. Spend all that money on organic foods. Don't drink too much caffiene. Make sure you test. Make sure there's a calculated bolus. Can't she have a break?

Internal Motivational Speaker: No! This is full time! Twenty-four hours a day. I work long hours, you know, Stomach. Some of us don't have the luxury of taking our time to digest!

Rocco looks at me with pleading eyes. I know, Rocco. I'm starving. Let's go downstairs and get a snack while they're arguing.

Stomach: Do you ever stop?

Internal Motivational Speaker: Does your mom ever stop?

Stomach: Don't you be bringing my mom into this!

Dollar clutched in my hand and leading Rocco by his chain, we sneak out. A few minutes later, I'm bolusing for the 25 grams of carbohydrate and Rocco is licking blueberry Nutrigrain crumbs off his paws.

Hungry

We went arrived at a film festival in Boston around 4 o'clock, after driving from Rhode Island. Hours later, I felt the churning, swirling ache in my stomach. That irritability and emptiness, making the railing of the theater's chair seem soft, and chewy.

"When did we eat last?" I whispered to Chris as the fifteenth short film started.

"At 3 o'clock."

My stomach rumbled.

"And what time is it now?"

"I don't know. Check your pump." Quick hit of the button to illuminate the screen. "It's 9:30."

A little bit shaky. Kind of weak. What was going on? I must be like 50 mg/dl. I pulled my meter from my purse and, by the backlight of my pump and meter, watched the countdown from 5 ... 4 ... 3 ... 2 ... 1 ...

174 mg/dl.

Not even resembling a low blood sugar. I bolused a unit to bring me back towards 100 mg/dl and sat back in my seat to watch the rest of the film. My stomach ached in protest. "Hey lady. Go eat something. It's been like seven hours. I'm empty."

Is this what hungry feels like?

Before I went on an insulin pump, I never really knew how "being hungry" felt. Back when I was using NPH and Lente and Ultra Lente insulins, I kept to an eating schedule that protected me from the peaks and valleys of my insulin. Even transitioning to Lantus had me eating on a scheduled basis, as the insulin seemed to peak a bit in my body. Going more than three hours without a little snack was unheard of.

Flash forward 17 years to making use of an insulin pump. At the age of 25, I started using my Paradigm 512 and it allowed me, for the first time in my life as a person with diabetes, to eat when I felt like it.

I could sleep until noon and not have to worry about blood sugar fluctuations. I could go to bed at three in the morning and my A1C didn't suffer the consequences. (Though the bags under my eyes were impressive.) And I didn't have to eat every three hours to ensure that my sugars would remain range-ish.

For the first time that I could remember, I felt "hungry." And the feeling was so new and startling yet familiar and uncomfortable that I couldn't help but associate it with being low.

We finally left the film festival and wandered towards the car. "Eat something," my stomach pleaded, lurching and trying to turn itself inside out.

"Let's eat," said Chris, almost in answer to my hungry belly.

"One quick thing," I murmured, reaching for my kit again. 144 mg/dl.

Hunger! I would have bet money on the fact that I was low.

Someone Else's Childhood

For Valentine's Day, Chris and I went to a French restaurant to celebrate our marriage and our growing family.

Since I'm seven months pregnant, we didn't crack open any bottles of wine during this dinner, but instead decided to indulge on a delicious fruit plate with chocolate fondue, with white chocolate and hazelnut dipping sauces on the side.

"What is this stuff?" I asked, easing my strawberry into the small dish of hazelnut spread.

"It's Nutella. You've never had that before?"

"No. It tastes like hazelnuts and sort of like chocolate. But it's not chocolate. And it's seriously awesome. What's it called again?" I couldn't stop rambling – this stuff was totally hitting the spot, appeasing my craving for something sweet and decadent.

"Nutella. You're being serious? You've never had this before?"

"Why would my mother ever introduce me to this sort of thing? I'd have stolen jars of it from the store and eaten them in one gulp, had I known." I smiled ruefully, thinking of the E.L. Fudge cookie binges I went on as a kid, rearranging the remaining cookies in the sleeve to hide the holes where the missing cookies had once been.

"Good point." He handed me another strawberry. "Bolus away."

I hadn't ever stuck a spoon into a jar of Fluff and gobbled up a few bites, and juice is not "for fun," but it's always for low blood sugars. It was strange to picture a childhood where Ring Dings weren't eaten in secret, or where rice cakes weren't used as barter in third grade for a Snicker's bar in the cafeteria. (For the record, no one ever wanted my rice cakes. They usually ended up shoved back into my book bag and eaten on the bus by this weird kid who also ate mud pies.)

Food is such a tricky, tricky thing for me, and enjoying a sweet treat in public isn't ever easy. I usually swallow a little bit of guilt with each bite of sweet, but I know that carrying the guilt isn't fair. If I'm respecting my diabetes control when I indulge, there's no harm in finding out just how delicious Nutella can be.

But when the check arrived, and with it, a wand of freshly spun, light pink cotton candy, I exclaimed excitedly, "Oooh! Cotton candy! I've only had that once before!"

Chris's face broke into a wide smile as I twirled off a small section of the spun sugar and tasted someone else's childhood.

In a Pickle

"You can eat any food you want, so long as it tastes like a pickle?" my daughter asked, looking excited.

"Not just pickle-flavored things, kiddo. But I can eat pickles without taking insulin because they are low in carbohydrates. Also cucumbers. And most of the stuff in a salad. And those wiggly Jell-O blobs we make sometimes."

Explaining the concept of "free foods" to my daughter was an exercise in borderline silliness because she is still learning about my diabetes, and she is only five years old. But the concept of healthy foods is not one we shy away from at home, and she has a strong grasp on what's a good choice versus a less nutritious one. Over the last year or so, Birdy and I have had conversations about how healthy food isn't just important for her mom because of diabetes, but that all people should be considering the food they eat carefully.

Discussions about how diabetes makes me think of things in sometimes special ways happen all the time between my daughter and I. Because she and I have been home together for the last five years, the daily duties of diabetes are commonplace for Birdy. She's seen me change countless pump sites, apply dozens of Dexcom sensors, and take boluses of insulin for hundreds of meals. Diabetes isn't something that's a big deal, but it's definitely pervasive in our life.

("Mom, where is your pump on your body? I don't want to bonk my head on it." Standard question these days, as my pump is usually clipped to my body at my daughter's eye level, leaving her head-butting into it every time she gives me a hug.) But lately, she's started to notice when I take out my pump and bang on the buttons and when I don't. And, because her curiosity is insatiable, she asks a ton of questions.

Which lead us to the discussion about free foods (after I clarified that the foods were free from carbs, but we still have to pay for them). I explained that there are a bunch of foods I can eat that I don't need to take insulin for because they are really low in carbs and don't have a lot of sugar in them. These foods are good to snack on when my blood sugar is a little high but I'm still hungry, because they won't make my number go even higher.

"They're the opposite of foods like pasta or cake, because those foods have lots of carbs and sugar in them and I need to take a lot of insulin for those."

"Right, except if you have a low blood sugar."

Maybe the discussion wasn't an exercise in silliness after all. Maybe it was more of a real-life lesson in the nuances of diabetes, the importance of food, and how you need to be aware of what you're eating.

"The free foods are ones that don't have as much sugar or crabs in them?"

"Carbs, baby."

"That's what I said."

Close enough.

Diabetes Food Lies

So many rules were slapped into place immediately upon diagnosis, with diabetes feeling like a disease of "don'ts." Don't eat cookies, don't forget to measure your food, don't leave the house without your meter or insulin or glucose tabs, don't go to bed without checking your blood sugar, don't eat too much sugar-free candy or else you will take up temporary yet violent residence in the bathroom.

But some of the don'ts were more subtle, like "don't allow the disease that's built around obsessing about food to let you become obsessed with food."

My mom used to hide packages of cookies in her closet, and I'd wait until she was in the shower to sneak into her walk-in and grab cookies by the fistful. I'd eat until my stomach ached and I didn't take an injection to cover my indulgences, and to this day, I still grapple with the "why" of my actions.

Guilt and food went hand-in-hand right away for me, as a kid with diabetes. I felt guilty about eating those closeted cookies, and even more guilty about lying to my mother about my actions.

And yet I did it anyway. I have a very clear memory of hiding a carton of ice cream underneath the couch upon hearing my father's approaching footsteps, afraid not of him telling me I couldn't eat it, but being angry that I didn't care enough to take insulin to cover it. I have no idea why I never bolused for those sneaky snacks; it was as if taking insulin for them forced me to acknowledge that I shouldn't have eaten it in the first place, as though the bolus itself made the action real, instead of the resulting high blood sugar. Or, you know, chewing and swallowing.

I never wanted to have that high blood sugar. I just didn't want to have the restrictions, and my way of rebelling against them seemed rooted in pretending I didn't have the rules of diabetes to own up to. Rebelling was so subtle, and so easy, for me.

Now, as an adult, I still find my feelings about food to be complicated. I feel very lucky that I have never dealt with a formalized eating disorder and I always accepted, even if I didn't always like, the shape and layout of my physical body, but diabetes has a way of making me view food through a lens that my non-diabetic friends don't share. My mind knew that numbers on the scale or the size tab on the back of my pants didn't matter as much as number on my meter, but still, it is always a struggle to remind myself of that fact.

The guilt that comes with my relationship with food, as a person living with type 1 diabetes, is always on my plate.

I live in my own house with my husband and my daughter, and I still have that urge to hide my food. Last night, I had an uncomfortable low blood sugar reaction that I decided to use the candy conversation hearts in the deli drawer of my fridge to treat, instead of glucose tabs, and as the deli drawer creaked as it slid open, I wondered if my husband thought I was just "sneaking candy." (For the record, Chris hasn't ever, ever made me feel guilty or judged for what I'm eating. The guilt isn't borne from the reaction of others, but from my own projected perceptions. It's a weird head game.) Some of the thoughts remain, but my mini-binges stopped long ago, once the don'ts of my mid-1980's diagnosis of type 1 diabetes gave way to today's modern insulins, meters, and mindsets.

A few days ago, a parent wrote to me and asked me why her child with type 1 diabetes would lie about eating certain foods. I had no idea what to say, because I still don't know why I did it myself, or why I still sometimes have the urge to do it. All I know is that even with a supportive family, friends who don't judge, access to like-pancreased people, and a mindset dominated by confidence in my diabetes management, I struggle to explain what made me binge-eat those cookies, or binge-lie about doing it. And I don't know why, decades later, it's still hard to say out loud.

Starting the Pump

The FedEx box loomed in the middle of the room.

Special overnight delivery. On a Saturday, no less. The room shrank as the box got bigger.

I made myself a cup of tea and sat down on the floor. Peeled back the packing tape. The flaps sprang open and a few stray foam peanuts flung themselves onto the floor, falling victim to Abby's big paws. Reaching into the box, I foraged around until I found the green, white and blue box inside. "Medtronic Minimed. Paradigm 512."

It looked like a pager. Slightly bigger, maybe, weighing in a just a few ounces. Smokey gray in color and almost transparent, I could see all the gears and wires inside.

Sipping my tea, I clipped it to the top of my shorts and stood up. I felt unbalanced, as though I would tip to one side if an aggressive breeze blew through. Leaving it attached, I jumped up and down.

Nothing happened. I sat on the couch to see if it I would feel its presence. I walked over to the window and looked out onto the deck, hearing the soft clink of the pump as it touched against the window sill.

The box of infusion sets was decidedly dodgier. Twenty-three inches of snaky, thin translucent tubing. The round white patch of gauze with the bright blue cap on it. A 6 mm cannula.

Prying open the infusion set packaging, I touched the tip of the needle with my finger. It was hollow and very sharp. I lifted up my shirt and exposed my stomach, daring myself to press the needle tip against my skin. It was as expected – sharp, but similar to the syringes I already used.

Syringes felt familiar. I'd used them many times a day for over seventeen years. Was I ready for this? This change? This whole new regimen?

I pressed the needle hard against my stomach, watching as my skin resisted, then that sliding *pop* of compliance as the needle embedded itself. I pulled out the blue cap and inspected the infusion set in my stomach for the first time. It looked like the cap on children's Tylenol. Like a tiny little pop-o-matic Trouble bubble on my abdomen.

Standing in front of the full-length mirror in my bathroom, the infusion set was bright white against my skin. I pulled my shirt tight over it and saw its outline against the fabric. It didn't hurt. It wasn't big. It could go unnoticed. My body still looked the same. I was still the same.

This small thing, clipped to my belt and the cannula under my skin, was going to help me achieve better control. It was going to assist me in lowering my otherwise plateaued A1C. The pump was going to afford me the freedom of sleeping late, conquering the dawn phenomenon, and bolusing teeny increments of insulin.

I felt different, though. This pump was the first external sign of my diabetes. And that, after 17 years of quiet injections and subtle finger pricks, stirred up the oddest combination of pride and fear. I have done this for so long, the only way I knew how. This new method was daunting. I had no idea that my A1C would drop within three months. Or that I would sleep late on a Saturday and not end up hypoglycemic. Or that I would feel strikingly healthier and confidently safer two years later.

I felt otherwise changed.

It was startling to look in the mirror and still see me.

Do You Like It?

"Excuse me ... your, um, arm? What's that on your arm?"

Ninety-five percent of the time, I don't care if people ask about my insulin pump or CGM. More power to them for being bold enough to embrace the awkwardness and actually ask, instead of assuming. (And even in the 5% moments of "argh – stop looking, don't ask," it usually ends up being a moment of discussion and disclosure for which I'm grateful.

"On my arm? That's my insulin pump. I have diabetes."

I was in line at the coffee shop, grabbing an iced coffee, escaping the blazing summer temperatures for a few minutes before heading back to work. I was wearing a skirt and a tank top, with my infusion set connected to the back of my right arm. My body – thanks to third trimester expansion, has run out of subtle places to stash my insulin pump, so it was casually clipped to the strap of my tank top.

Kind of noticeable, but in a "who cares" sort of way. It's hot outside. And I'm wicked pregnant. And I have no waist anymore. You can see my insulin pump? Good for you. You can probably see my belly button, too.

"No kidding. Diabetes? Is it because of the pregnancy?"

"No, I've had diabetes way longer than this pregnancy. I was diagnosed when I was seven."

The guy paused for a second, his eyes lingering on the infusion set on my arm. "So you do that thing instead of shots?"

"Yep."

"Do you like it?"

That question always throws me a little. Do I like it? The pump? I do like the pump. I like not taking injections. I like not whipping out syringes at the dinner table and exposing my skin. I like taking tiny bits of insulin to correct minor highs. I like running temp basals to beat back hypos. I like people wondering what it might be instead of assuming it's a medical device.

"I do like it. It works for me." I paused, already envious of the coffee in his hand. "I like coffee more, though."

He laughed and finished paying for his coffee. "Can't blame you for that. Good luck with the baby, and try to stay cool in this weather," he said.

I don't like diabetes. That's a certainty. It is exhausting and I'm burnt out on the demands it places on my life. But the pump? Yes, I do like it. It's a streamlined delivery mechanism for a hormone I wish my body would just cave and start making again. It handles diabetes so I can go back to trying to put my socks on without tipping over.

Why I Pump

It took me years to use an insulin pump. Actual years. I was on multiple daily injections for 17 years before deciding to take the cyborg plunge, and honestly, it's one of the best decisions I've made in terms of making sense of my diabetes.

I use an insulin pump because it keeps me from having blood sugar bumps in the wee hours of the morning (thank you, dawn phenomenon). I'm able to correct mild hyperglycemia with a precise dose of insulin. Unless I forget to reattach my insulin pump after showering (which has only happened to me once in 15+ years of pumping but now that I've typed that sentence it will happen to me every day for a year), I always have insulin on me. I really prefer changing an infusion set every three days versus taking seven to nine injections a day.

My decision to use an insulin pump is reinforced every time I take a short pump break. Disconnecting from my devices is nice for the first few hours because of the novelty and my body's ability to be unadorned for just a bit. But yeah, then that novelty wears off and I'm immediately annoyed with the need to remember to stick an insulin pen in my bag and the piercing of my skin every few hours and the bruising left behind by each injection. After a day or two, I remember why basal rate changes are powerful and why precision dosing of my insulin is effective.

And I'm amazed by the progress I've seen in the last 15 years, especially with hybrid-closed loop system running on my insulin pump right now. Looking back at my 24-hour pump graph and seeing the red lines indicating that my basal rate has shut off to help ward off a low blood sugar ... man, that is amazing. My low blood sugars have lessened in severity and frequency as a result of a machine doing the "thinking" for me.

I'm able to pump because my insurance company and my job make access to this technology easier. I pump because it makes my diabetes more convenient. I wear this pump because it helps me keep my blood sugars in a range that makes me feel pretty good.

I pump because I don't make any of my own damn insulin and wearing this little device helps turn down the back burner of diabetes busy-brain. And that is a big win in my daily scuffle with this disease.

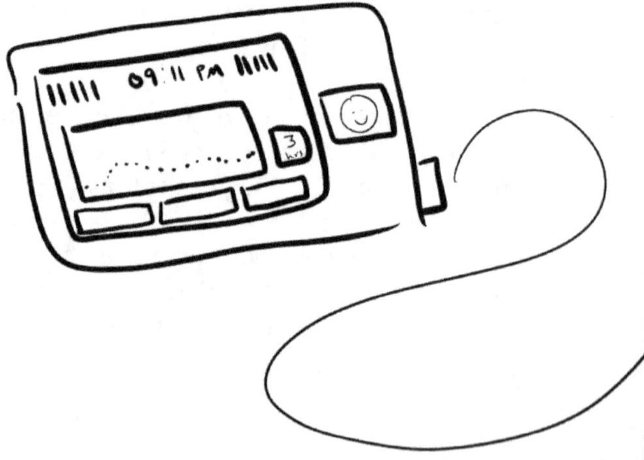

Rage Bolus

October 10, 2005: Bit of a rantish post here. And there's no reason for this other than to vent frustration.

Last night, after I came home from the U2 show in Boston, I was a little bit high. Rang in at 212 mg/dl. Okay, no problem. Bolus it up, go to bed. Woke up this morning at 200 mg/dl. Hmmm, no drop in the blood sugar levels. Not to worry, though, because today is infusion set change day. Pump primed and new infusion set inserted. I set about dressing for work.

Arrived at work. Hungry. Devoured one of those sometimes-delicious-but-most-often-just-gritty Kashi Whole Grain Granola bars. Bolused two units to cover, in accordance with the 1:10 ratio. Worked at my boring job for about an hour before realizing that I had already visited the bathroom twice in that time. Hmmm. Not normal. Tested, revealing 281 mg/dl. Whaaaa... I corrected this morning. I bolused for the crappy snack. And now I'm higher than before? Frustrated Kerri. So I rage bolus*. I just crank the shit out the pump, knowing full well that I only need about two units to come back down. I send in 3.5 units. Sit back, satisfied.

Not done yet. I test again, an hour and half later, clocking in at 286 mg/dl. Fan-freaking-tastic. Good thing all that insulin made me higher. Because that makes sense. So I rage bolus again, sending two more units coursing through, Frustrated Kerri not really giving a shit that the active insulin tally on my pump is enough to cover dinner at Olive Garden.

So it's noon. I've been high all morning. I just changed my infusion set this morning. And I'm angry. I do not want to pull this set only to find that it's perfectly fine and I've wasted yet another expensive pump supply.

I'm riding this out. It's Me against the D. Who will persevere? How high will Kerri allow herself to rise before she pulls the set and starts over? How much rage bolusing will eventually catch up with Herself before Kerri bottoms out at 44 mg/dl? How many licks does it indeed take to reach the center of a Tootsie Roll Tootsie Pop? (Not three. It at least takes 125.)

I'm going to find out as soon as my rage bolusing catches up with me and I'm trick-or-treating at people's desks here at work.

** Rage Bolus: Taking an uncalculated amount of insulin to correct a frustrating high blood sugar reading*

Disco Boobs

Over the holidays, my husband and I had the opportunity to join his agent, who happened to be in town, for dinner. Grown-up time, sans BSparl. I wore tights. It was a fancier than our average Tuesday night.

So we all sat down to dinner and while everyone was talking, I reached into my purse to do a quick blood sugar check and to remote bolus for the bread and olive oil that had been placed on the table. My hands stirred up the contents of my purse, but didn't score the meter.

"Damn, I know exactly where it is," I mumbled to myself, picturing my meter case on the front seat of our car, which was down the street and tucked into a parking lot.

Conveniently, I had this scrappy little One Touch Mini rolling around in my purse, so I was able to test, but I was out of luck in the remote bolusing department. And with my pump tucked discreetly, but snuggly, into the front of my bra (clip against my sternum, buttons on the pump facing out), it wasn't exactly the most readily available medical device. Not without some seriously awkward self-groping, that is.

Chris was watching me scramble. "Just pull your napkin up and grab your pump. No one will notice," he whispered.

"You don't think I should excuse myself to the ladies' room?"

"Nah, go for it."

So while everyone was talking, I reached down the front of my dress and deftly grabbed my insulin pump. I programmed in the bolus and then went to tuck it back into my outfit without anyone noticing.

Except.

Once you've begun a bolus on the Animas pump, if you press a button while that bolus is administering, it prompts the pump to cancel the bolus. It's a great safety feature for when you realize, mid-bolus, that you absolutely do NOT want to take five units of Humalog to cover a spinach salad. But it's not so awesome when you accidentally hit a button while securing the pump to the front of your bra, and it suddenly starts singing a loud song. And lighting up, providing a strange glow from your chest, not unlike a medicinal disco ball.

"What's that?" One of our dinner companions asked, looking in my direction but not knowing the noise was coming from my body.

"Sounds like a cell phone!" One of the other dinner guests said, smiling and reaching for another piece of bread.

During the brief distraction, I snagged the pump again and programmed the bolus a second time, then stuck the pump back where it came from without issue.

"Oh, it's me. No big deal – all set now. So as we were saying ..." I felt the bolus going in, and the pump was quiet again. No need for me to get into a big explanation of "Oh, this is my INSULIN PUMP and I'm DIABETIC and YES I CAN EAT THE BREAD." It wasn't what I wanted to talk about that night. I just wanted to move on, and swiftly.

No one asked any questions, and the night went on to be a very nice one, with excellent food and great company.

And Chris and I definitely laughed our faces off when we got in the car to go home.

"So do you think your agent and his family think I have some kind of musical ... disco boobs?"

Toss 'Em in the Big Blue Hole

Am I a crumb because I want to rip my devices off sometimes and throw them into a great, blue hole? Like that one near Belize City? My skin is so irritated by the adhesives and intrusions of my insulin pump and my CGM that the desire to heave them into this abyss is intense.

I hate the bulk of them. The amount of room that my devices take up on my body and the trauma they have a tendency to leave on my skin. I simultaneously absolutely love the convenience of them. The fact that I can take precise doses of insulin without using a magnifying glass on a syringe or when the alarm goes off in the middle of the night, alerting me to a 70 mg/dL that was sliding towards LOW ... this is the stuff that makes wearing diabetes devices worth it for me.

The pros outweigh the cons by a long shot, but the cons are a thorn in my side these days. Or, more accurately, a relentless itch on my skin.

I took my insulin pump off one morning because the site was so sore, and so red, and the mark it left on my body was like a little diabetes bullet wound. I have a high threshold for irritation and itch, but this site was terrible and after pulling it out, I didn't have anything even close to resembling the desire to put a new one back in. I went on injections for 12 hours before realizing that being on the road wasn't doing my blood sugars any favors (I was having trouble bringing myself back under 200 mg/dL – rage bolus, anyone?), so once my Levemir injection timed out, I reluctantly put a new pump site in. Admittedly, blood sugar control for me these days is better on the pump.

It's not just my pump sites that are irritating these days. This morning, I noticed that my CGM site had become red, itchy, and irritated OUTSIDE OF THE TAPE.

Usually, I have a skin response underneath where the sensor actually is, or where any of the tapes connect. But this round, I have a proximity rash thanks probably to continuously compromised skin. So now I'm getting a frigging rash in the places where the sensor isn't even touching?! I'm in a hard place of feeling safer with access to CGM data but access to CGM data produces a fierce itch.

I need a breather. But taking one leaves me exposed. HEAVE this shit into the great blue hole! That's what I'm doing mentally, chucking all these things that make my skin hurt and itch into the watery hole and watching them sink to the bottom.

... but then diving in to rescue them. Because I hate injections and I hate going to bed without seeing my CGM trend arrow.

How to Have Sex with an Insulin Pump

Don't. For the love of God, do not have sex with your insulin pump. It's an expensive insulin delivery device, and it's not to be trifled with.

But if the Google search you made was to find out how to have sex with the insulin pump *in the vicinity*, then that's a whole different take. Because that topic comes up a lot in the women's discussion groups that I've taken part in, and it was a particularly hot topic at a conference I attended. The same sorts of questions come up every time, from new pumpers and people considering adding a diabetes device to their management plan:

"How do you deal with wearing a device when you're trying to be, like, naked?"

"Do you disconnect during intimacy?"

"Does it get in the way, physically?"

"Does it get in the way, emotionally?"

For the record, I love that these questions get asked. And the best part is, they're asked in rooms full of women who have either met for the first time that day or haven't even formally met yet. Diabetes, for all its chaos, does bring a certain level of discussion comfort and camaraderie, and I couldn't love that more.

"How do you deal with wearing a device when you're trying to be, like, naked?"

This was a tough hurdle for me, because I went so long without wearing any devices.

Diagnosed as a kid and not pumping until 2004 or CGM'ing until 2006, I spent a big part of my diabetes life without any external "symptoms," so to speak. Initially, I needed to be comfortable with my device(s) before I could expect anyone else to be, and that did take some time.

But I like the "no big deal" philosophy to these moments. If I give the impression that these devices aren't a big deal and should be taken as a small part of the bigger whole, then I hope my partner will follow suit. For the most part, wearing a pump and a CGM isn't something I feel self-conscious about, but being honest, there are days when I want to rip them both off and throw them across the room in pursuit of feeling truly naked. I don't like having these artificial bits and pieces stuck to me all the time, but I try to keep tabs on the bigger picture, which is my overall health.

Sounds cheesy, but it's the truth.

"Do you disconnect during intimacy?"

Personally, I do. I don't like having anything connected to me during those moments, because it becomes a distraction. I like feeling like diabetes is a back burner issue in the bedroom, or at least as much of one as I manage. When I first started pumping, disconnecting felt awkward because I didn't know how to make it feel sexy ("Oh, let me just slip out of my medical device and into something more comfortable," never had the right tone to it.) and it took me out of the mood a little bit.

But once I was comfortable pumping, in all capacities, I was comfortable with this part, too. Disconnecting is kind of like my mating call now, which is a bit strange but also 'no big deal.'

"Does it get in the way, physically?

Not for me, because I'm already disconnecting. And I take care to keep my devices as out-of-the-way as I can manage, keeping infusion sets on the back of my hip and sensors on my thighs, leaving my abdomen feeling "normal." Sometimes it gets in the way in the initial moments, like when it's being disconnected and I'm trying to figure out where to stash it for the time being (bedside table? under a pillow? on the floor? It's a tough device, but I'm not willing to throw a six-thousand-dollar medical device onto the floor with reckless abandon.), but for the most part, once it's disconnected, I forget about it. The trouble is sometimes remembering to reconnect afterwards. Some women set the alarm on their pump to remind them, but I'm not even close to that organized. Others set reminders on their phone. I've never gone to bed without reconnecting, so I'm going to pretend that I will always remember?

"Does it get in the way, emotionally?"

Yes, at least enough so that I can't outright say no. Can't lie – not being able to be completely naked (sans pump site and CGM transmitter, for me) is a weird feeling, and I always feel like I need to give Chris a head's up as to where my devices are currently connected. "Be careful of the site on my right arm," or "sensor is on the left," sort of directions feel anti-intimacy, for me. But that's where the relationship with my husband comes into play – he makes me feel like diabetes is something we can openly discuss, so it makes device topography easier to disclose, knowing he's not creeped out by this stuff. The emotions about this sort of thing ebb and flow, just like emotions about diabetes in general, but it's most important for me to be able to talk about it with Chris. Being part of a team that allows for the emotional highs and lows helps keep devices from getting in the way, mentally.

You can have sex with your insulin pump ... by your side. Or on the bedside table. Intimacy with diabetes requires a little forethought in addition to the foreplay (terrible pun), but it can be done. Just don't shag your actual pump, or you could end up with a different set of issues entirely.

Highs and Lows

Highs and Lows

Going through SixUntilMe.com, I found many essays about low blood sugars. Hypoglycemic episodes make for "good stories" because most people with insulin-dependent diabetes have had a nasty low, and sharing those stories forges a bond.

My low blood sugars have changed over the years. When I was young, my blood sugars were closely monitored by my parents, but NPH and Regular insulins made for serious peaks and valleys of control. Some of the most debilitating lows came in my early 20's, when I would feel the waves of unconsciousness lapping at me. Thankfully, low blood sugars are less frequent and less severe these last few years; a credit to the technology I am lucky to access.

What struck me about this collection is that it's mostly lows, with few mentions about high blood sugars. And that's not because they are less frequent or less intense. They just made for less acute narratives. And now, years after I stopped writing my website, I realized that highs are often partnered with character assassinations. Highs are met with "What did you eat?" or "What did you do to cause this high?" Judgment about hypoglycemia feels less accusatory than judgments about highs.

It's funny, how highs and lows come loaded with emotions. Aren't they just data points? Isn't that what our clinical teams tell us? Just a bunch of numbers to guide decisions?

Then why are there so many feelings attached to those numbers?

A Jacket, Just in Case

BEEP BEEP BEEP

2 am

Low alarm. Where am I?

Hotel.

Hotel room in Kansas City.

Damp. Damp with sweat. My long sleeve shirt stuck to the inside of my elbows, ironed by panic.

BEEP BEEP BEEP

Kansas City. That's where I am. Why am I beeping?

51 mg/dL. That red circle with the down arrow attached to it.

Asking to be calibrated.

Meter check. 32 mg/dL.

BEEP BEEP BEEP

No fucking way am I in the 30s. I start to come around a little bit, taking the six tabs left in my glucose tab jar and chewing them all at once, unhinging my jaw like a snake.

Prick finger again. Test strip.

31 mg/dL

Think fast. Unsure if I have enough tabs to correct this low blood sugar. Even if I do, unsure if they will hit fast enough. Felt swimmy in the brain. Can't pass out in this room. No one will know for hours.

Quick decisions made. Pull on sneakers. Grab cell phone and room key.

Walk to the hotel room door. Open it.

Wait, if I pass out, I want to have a jacket on.

(WHY?)

Put my jacket over my pajamas. Sprint to hotel elevator, reasoning the adrenaline will help boost my number? Sweating like I've run a marathon instead of just down the hall.

Downstairs. Took 30 seconds. Felt like 3 hours.

BEEP BEEP BEEP

Walked to the hotel sundries shop near the check in desk. I saw juice and snacks when I checked in. Grab an orange juice. Drank it in one long pull while standing at the cooler. Grab another orange juice.

My face felt confused, like my mouth had slid down into my neck. Also completely lucid, despite plummeting blood sugar and migrating facial features.

Hotel concierge.

"Hi, how can I help you?"

I look drunk. Or lost. Or both.

Low, though.

Not sure what I said. I know I said diabetes and low blood sugar and I'm sorry fifteen times. I told him my full name, maybe more than once. That I was embarrassed but was afraid I would pass out in my room so I thought I'd be safer in the lobby. "I put my jacket on just in case I passed out!" Laughed too loudly at my own not-a-joke.

He calmly sat me down on a couch in the lobby and unwrapped candies from the hotel's leftover trick-or-treat stash, leaving them open-faced but still on the wrapper, lined up on the hotel bench like breadcrumbs to bring me back to myself.

BEEP BEEP BEEP

"Are you feeling better?"

I wasn't sure. My hands were shaking a whole lot. But I could feel the hypo fog starting to lift and I knew it was going to be okay in a few minutes. His coworkers came over and lingered casually but carefully, standing over the lady in her pajamas with her jacket on, trick-or-treating a few days too late in the lobby.

Eventually, it was fine. Embarrassing and humbling but fine. I was grateful that someone was willing to sit with a stranger while her blood sugar tumbled, then climbed.

The hotel employee's name is written on a post-it note in my jacket pocket. With his manager's email. And the contact information for their corporate office.

The gift basket I am sending this guy is going to be epic.

Disclosures

"Do you guys have any fun plans for the summer?"

The question was simple enough, but not even close to a level my hypoglycemia-addled brain could handle. I had trouble formulating a response, and the lag time was embarrassing. We've only moved to the neighborhood a few months ago and haven't solidified relationships with our neighbors yet, so being wickedly low in front of someone new wasn't my favorite way to disclose my diabetes.

Thankfully, a disclosure had already happened, to a certain extent. When she had asked me about my work travel this past week and what I did for work, I said that I worked in patient advocacy and that I'd had diabetes since I was a kid. She nodded in recognition and shared that her college roommate was also T1D, so my disclosure was pleasantly subtle and streamlined. No big deal. What I hadn't anticipated was going low during the course of our conversation.

And I was low. Wickedly low. The kind of low that made my face feel like it was full of Novocain and that my hands were like fish out of water at my sides, twitching and flapping absently.

I scanned the trees in the front yard for some kind of hint.

"Pssssst. You guys! You, trees! Do I have fun plans for the summer?"

They only waved their leaves at me. "We have no idea! Go get something to eat, dummy!"

"We go to Maine. MAINE." I said it twice with way too much emphasis on the second one, an angry seal barking out their summer plans.

My neighbor didn't seem to notice that my eyes weren't able to focus on her, and I'm fairly certain she didn't hear my Dexcom receiver hollering at me from the front steps of the house. But I knew that another minute or two was the chasm between attempted conversation and calling for medical help, so I had to embrace the awkward.

"I'm so sorry; I know I mentioned that I have diabetes and you said your college roommate also had diabetes. So I'm really, really low at the moment and I need to go inside to grab some juice. Would you excuse me for a minute?" I was trying to be polite and not let on that my thoughts were knocking around in my head like socks in a dryer. She nodded and I took off for the kitchen, where I downed a glass of grape juice as quickly as I could.

My CGM only told me I was "LOW" and I cursed myself for not responding faster to the beeping.

Coming back outside, we stepped back into conversation without much pause, watching our kids play in the front yard.

"Sorry about that," I said. "No problem at all," she warmly responded, not missing a beat.

And I kept an eye on my CGM graph, watching my blood sugars rise and kindly deposit thoughts back into my head.

Emergency Plan

Was just 106 mg/dL. Tumbled fast to 40.

Took minutes. Felt like seconds.

Dizzy.

Wait – get phone.

Put the baby in his crib.

He's safe in there.

Already drank juice – plenty of it – now wait wait waaaaaaaait.

…. Waaaaaaiting.

Wall edges seem wiggly, like if I poked them, they'd shudder like Jell-O.

Baby is safely in the crib, giggling and playing with his feet. I sit on his floor with my phone in my hand, ready to make a phone call to a neighbor if the waves of confusion start to erode my mental shore.

Briefly wonder what I'd say if I called. "Hey, this is Kerri. Can you come over? I feel like I'm going to pass out." I'm sure I'd try to sound casual when casual is not how I feel. I keep 911 dialed so if I need to just hit the call button, I'm ready.

Emergency plans. I have them.

My tongue becomes less thick, less clumsy in my mouth. I flex my fingers, which are attached to my still-shaking hands. They feel responsive but like their wings are still clipped.

Juice starts to change the course of my blood sugar. CGM alarms still blaring from my phone, less urgently now. Walls seem less gelatinous.

Baby burps and then laughs at his own burp. I laugh, too, the fog of hypoglycemia unwrapping from around my brain. I remember that it's morning. That it's a week day. That I'm due on a conference call in 20 minutes.

CGM shows me a comforting arrow.

Emergency over. Status quo returned.

Before I retrieve the baby from his crib, I grab a cloth and clean up the juice that leapt from the glass while my hands were birds.

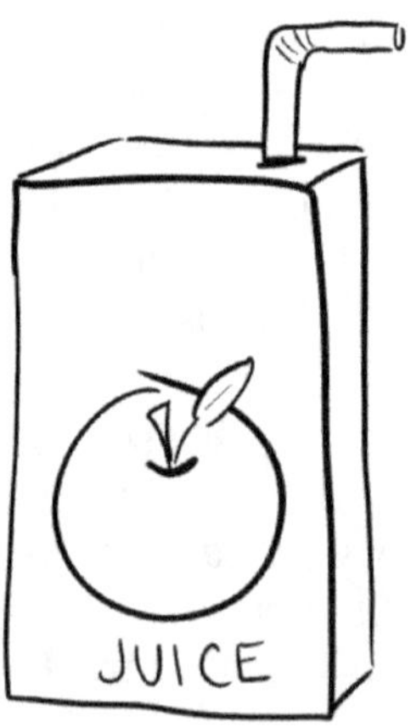

Employee of the Month

Yesterday at lunch, I was browsing at one of my favorite stores and picking through a pile of spring sweaters. (Buy one, get one 50% off! I'm a sucker for a good sale.) I find two sweaters that are pretty and springy and have that nice, soft cottony feel that you want to rub against your cheek.

Then those feelings hit. The ones where my jacket felt warm and heavy against the spring chill but suddenly made me feel like it was a fabric tanning booth - too hot, too heavy, and like the sleeves were thick with mud.

"Excuse me? I know it's a weird question, but do you have any juice or candy in this store?"

When will I learn to put my glucose tabs into my purse? Here's hoping that happens soon.

The pregnant woman behind the counter gave me an odd look. "I don't ... hang on ... um, I have half of a mini Milky Way bar? Is that okay? You just hungry, sweetie?"

"No." My tongue was too big for my mouth, making it hard to talk. "Can I just leave these here for a few minutes? I'll be right back."

Walking with determined, focused steps, I went outside to where my car was parked and unlocked the door. Leaning in the passenger side, I grabbed the bottle of glucose tabs from the center console.

"Damn it, two? Only two are in here?" The bottle was almost empty, save for two lonely glucose tabs. I poured them into my hands and ate them at the same time, the glucose tab dust coming out and snowing all over the passenger seat of my car.

"Gee whiz," I said. (What's that? Not kidding you on that one? Fine. I dropped an F bomb right there, outside of a sweater shop.) I noticed a Panera Bread next door so I slammed my car door and walked over there, listening to the Dexcom blaring from inside my purse.

There was a line for lunch. Four cashiers were working furiously, but the low was creeping up just as fast and my legs were beginning to buckle.

"I need orange juice. I'm diabetic and having a low blood sugar. Can you please help me as quickly as you can?" I stood there in my work clothes and my coat, with my grown-up purse over my arm and started to cry because I couldn't function properly and I was becoming more and more confused. Not sobbing, not whining, not outwardly breaking down, but big tears rolled out of my eyes without permission and headed for my jawline.

The boy behind the counter was taken aback. "Stay here. Stand here. I'll be right back. Don't move." He ran and returned with a glass of juice. I moved toward him like one of those koi fish in a park pond, fighting for crumbs of bread.

He watched as I drank the entire glass without stopping, knowing that people in line were watching me and staring and I couldn't bring myself to care.

"You good? You seem better already, right?" CounterBoy answered his own question. "You're good. You're fine."

I fumbled with my wallet. "How much do I owe you?"

"Miss, it's okay. I'm happy to pay for that orange juice myself. Please."

"No, I'm diabetic but I have a job. And I appreciate your help." The Novocain of the low was starting to wear off a bit, just by knowing the juice was in my system. "I'd really like to pay."

"Okay, let's just call it a small, okay? That's a dollar. A dollar is fine." He punched the keys of the register. "$1.05" came up on the digital screen.

"A dollar five. Okay." I handed him a dollar and dug around in my pocket for a nickel. "Here you go. Exact change. We're good."

He put the money in the register and wiped his forehead with his wrist. "You sure you're okay? Do you want to sit for a minute?" A guy waiting in line mumbled something about 'flirting on your own time.' CounterBoy raised an eyebrow. "Sir, this is a medical emergency. I just saved her life. Your sandwich? Little less important at the moment, okay?"

He turned back to me. "You good?"

"I'm good. Thank you for your help. I really appreciate it. You saved the day, man."

"I did. I saved the day." He squared his shoulders. "I'm going to be employee of the month!"

Bullets

The confusion is instant - the raw and palpable confusion where you know you're in trouble, but you haven't yet grasped just how much.

"FAILED SENSOR" on the Dexcom screen, and instead of reaching for the jar of glucose tabs, I reach down past my waistband and pull the Dexcom sensor free from my right thigh. It's stubborn; it wants to stay stuck and takes a firm pull to remove. The sticky residue left behind by the adhesive tape is in that familiar oval shape, and it grabs my fingers. I linger there for a minute, feeling the leftover glue securing to my thumb. I wonder how long this sensor would have stayed stuck if it hadn't FAILED.

The hotel heat vent switches on, which must explain the sweat on my forehead and in the crook of my elbow. My hands are trembling. I have diabetes. It's like a light bulb that goes off on my head, reminding me that I need to eat something. Sweat collects in a damp veil on my forehead and I wipe at it absently with the sleeve of my shirt. I slow-motion swat at the bottle of glucose tabs on the bedside table, counting out five ... six ... seven glucose tabs and holding them in my hand like magic beans.

My mouth isn't even mine. It's just this thing, this portal to shove giant sugar tablets into. I can't work up the saliva to chew, so the tab sits in my mouth until it starts to dissolve a little, and then my body remembers what to do with it. "Chew the damn thing."

Tragedy of a low - no saliva. Nothing to help mince these tabs down into something useful.

While chomping down on the fifth glucose tab, I test my blood sugar and see a 24 mg/dL on the meter. My first thought: "What a screwed-up number." There isn't a second thought.

No room. My focus is limited to chew, swallow, and stay awake. I feel the waves of consciousness lapping, and I find myself chewing in rhythm with the ocean in my mind.

Adrenaline kicks in and I'm suddenly aware of everything: the whirring of the hotel heating unit, the sounds of New York City waking up outside the window, the bottle of water on the bedside table, and the fact that my bangs are plastered messily to the side of my face, anchored by sweat and panic.

The second thought finally kicks in. "You're fine. You'll be fine. Seven glucose tabs ... you'll be over 100 soon and get on with things." It's an internal pep talk, running on a loop in my brain.

I shouldn't have had the wine the night before. I am angry at the sensor for dying after only four days. I wish I had set an alarm for 3 am to double-check my blood sugar. So many things. But mostly, I'm relieved, relieved, relieved because I felt the whoosh of the bullet as it went by.

Jet Lagged

I was on a plane, high above the clouds, looking down onto the world below me where everything looks too small and too distant to be affected by a number. Cruising altitude.

I felt his hand on my shoulder, shaking me a little bit.

"Kerri. Kerri, wake up. You're really sweaty. Wake up."

Was it the captain speaking? No, it was my fiancé. I was half-draped off the edge of the bed, pulling the long-sleeved blue t-shirt away from my body. The space above my collarbone was damp. My hands went to it, blotting it with my sleeve.

"I'm awake." I could hear my own voice but it sounded like it was coming from the end of a long tube of Christmas wrapping paper. "I'm going to test."

I unzipped the meter case, lanced the end of my finger, and watched as "39 mg/dl - do you need a snack?" popped up on the screen.

Everything was nonchalant and dreamy. "I'm 39."

Chris sprang from the bed and returned in just a few seconds with a glass of grape juice.

I drank it down in a few gulps, being careful not to let any spill out. "I'm pretty low. I don't feel that low." The words sounded so matter-of-fact, like we were discussing the thread count of our sheets.

"Did the thing go off?" He motioned to the CGM as he rescued the empty glass from my unsteady hands. I reached down for my pump and clicked a few buttons.

"No. It says I'm 74 mg/dl. But it's showing this crazy sharp dip - see, right there? - so it knows I'm dropping."

"Feeling better yet?"

"Not yet. I changed my site before we went out tonight. That always happens - I change my site, I end up higher, and the correction bolus crashes me down so hard." This conversation is happening as my blood sugar hovers around 40 mg/dl. Aren't people supposed to be on the cusp of a coma or something at this point? How is my brain busy explaining the mechanics of this crisis? Where is the SkyMall catalog? I'm still mid-flight on this low.

I clicked off the lamp and we both settled back into bed. As my blood sugar rose, I felt increasingly worse, shivering and cloudy-mouthed, my mind racing and my hands clenching against threats unseen. I felt like I was landing now. But the closer I came to landing on the safety of the ground, the more terrifying it became until the landing gear in my mind touched down and I was okay. Safe at 130 mg/dl.

The alarm went off this morning - my blood sugar was 119 mg/dl. I collected my baggage from the night before and rubbed the sleep from my eyes.

Today, I'm feeling a bit jet-lagged.

Lunchtime Lows

I'm standing at the counter at the bank and I hear my cell phone buzzing. Then I hear the Dexcom wailing out its BEEEEEEEP. My pump starts to buzz from inside my bra. Every bit of technology I have is exploding all at once and I'm just trying to make a damn deposit.

"Miss, I just need your account number."

"Account number, sure. I can get that for you." BEEEEEEEEP again. Why is it beeping again? It should only beep once when I'm high. My goodness, I'm awfully warm, despite standing underneath the bank air conditioning unit.

I stick my hand into my bag and forage about. My fingertips feel like they're trapped in cotton balls and I can't quite get a good handle on my wallet. Instead, I grab the Dexcom receiver, which is BEEEEEPing again, and press a button.

Oh shit, LOW. Below 40 mg/dl. I press the down button and see "39 mg/dl" next to the blood sugar graph, which now looks like the Cliffs of Insanity from The Princess Bride.

"Here is my license. Can you pull my account numbers by looking up my name, please? I'm diabetic and having a little low blood sugar at the moment and I need to drink this juice." I hand the teller my license and raise up the bottle of juice with my other hand, like one of the Price is Right models.

"No problem. I'll get your account numbers. Do you want to have a seat?"

"No, no thanks." I drain the bottle between words. "I'm good. I just need a minute to let my blood sugar come up."

He typed some numbers in on his keyboard and passed my receipt through the bank printer. "This isn't some elaborate plan to rob the bank, is it?"

I laughed. Just drinking the juice alleviated the low-panic enough for me to act like a normal (slightly sweaty) person.

"I'm not robbing the bank. But I may take one of those free lollipops, if that's okay."

He hands me my receipt, along with three purple lollipops. "Here you go. Why don't you wait a few minutes over there," he gestures towards the bank reception area, "for your blood sugar to come up? I don't want you to drive yet."

"Okay. Thanks for your help."

And I teeter carefully on my far-too-high-for-such-a-low heels over to one of the plush, blue chairs. Sinking into the chair and waiting for the juice to do its thing, I unwrapped one of the lollipops. My feet didn't quite reach the floor, as I was sitting so far back in the chair.

But I was starting to feel better.

People came in and out of the bank over the next ten minutes while I rested, looking over and most likely wondering what that grown woman was doing there, face flushed, swinging her feet, and sucking happily on a lollipop.

Sad Robot

I was 48 mg/dl after dinner.

I thought I had over-estimated a bit for dinner and when his words started swimming in the foreground before they slammed into my ears, my hands unzipped the black meter case without thinking. Grape juice stained my mouth but the moment ended with a sheepish smile and the admission that, "I think I over-bolused a little at dinner."

Before bed, I was 107 mg/dl. Safe. I curled against Chris, said a silent prayer for the cat to remain off my pillow, and fell asleep.

At 4:07 am, I woke up with the lamp on.

Then I remembered that I had woken up about 20 minutes earlier and turned the lamp on, like I was trying to wake up in stages. Shirt was wet and wilted against my skin, my face was cold with sweat. My meter case was open and lying next to me, but I couldn't remember testing.

Siah hopped up on the bed and purred loudly.

Moonlit lows had been leaving me alone lately, letting me cling to the few hours of sleep I was able to catch. But this one must have been hiding under the bed, knowing full well that my earlier low had sapped my liver of its glucagon storage. My thoughts were unraveling like a scarf. Did I test earlier?

Chris stirred next to me. For some reason, I was determined to let him sleep. I pressed the "on" button on the meter to recall the last result, my brain stuck in a routine of "test, then treat," even though I knew with every breath that I needed juice now.

Last result was the 107 mg/dl before bed.

Click. 5 ... 4 ... 3 ...

Siah put her little gray nose over the meter screen and pawed at my wrist.

42 mg/dl.

Nodding to myself almost matter-of-factly, I swung my shaking legs over the side of the bed and put my feet on the floor. I felt like I was made of yarn. My feet wouldn't plant themselves in place but instead they kept staggering, one after the other, throwing me into the wall. I tried to take a step forward and my knees buckled.

My brain is fully functioning. I know words. I know sounds. I know exactly what I need to do and what the number 42 means but my body has betrayed me and won't move as I have asked, like I was a robot who had been over-oiled.

Crawling back into the bed, I meant to tap Chris on the shoulder but instead my hand took on a force of its own and whacked him solidly in the chest.

"Help me?"

He woke up instantly.

"Sit down." In a matter of seconds, he was back with a bottle of juice, despite the fact that there were two juice bottles resting on the bedside table. Autopilot for both of us.

Again with the grape juice. Wiped my shirt against my forehead. He held my arm and kept me steady.

Drained the bottle. Zipped up the meter case. Routines, routines, robotic routines. Turned off the lamp. Collapsed against my pillow and listened to the sound of my labored breathing, aware of the hurricane of juice in my stomach and the tears in my eyes even though I didn't feel sad. I just felt low.

"It's okay. You're okay."

And I lay there, at the bottom of the well but slowly making the mechanical moves of resurfacing from that pit, like a sad robot. Wishing I could tell him "I know," but instead these tears fell out and my metal mouth wouldn't make the words.

Seven Versions of a Low Blood Sugar

SCENARIO: A blood sugar of 53 mg/dL caused me to wake up at 2 am, drink a juice box, and stay awake until 2.30 am waiting for my blood sugar to rise.

DESCRIBING TO MY FRIEND: "Yeah, sometimes diabetes is a thing at night. I had a low last night that woke me up around 2 am, but that's why I keep juice on the bedside table. Do you want coffee? I totally could use some coffee."

DESCRIBING TO MY HUSBAND: "Did you hear my alarm last night? Yeah, the juice box was from that. I need to make sure to grab the straw wrapper off the floor before the baby finds it. We need to buy more juice boxes, as I think that was the last one."

DESCRIBING TO MY MOTHER: "I was 53 mg/dL, but I had a juice box right there on the bedside table, and my CGM alarm woke me up, and I wasn't even tired this morning! No worries, Ma."

DESCRIBING TO MY INSURANCE COMPANY: "My continuous glucose monitor alarmed, waking me up at 2 am in time to treat a hypoglycemic event before encountering a seizure or similar. The glucagon kit in my bedside table was my last line of defense. This is why access to, and reimbursement for these tools is so important to me."

DESCRIBING TO SOMEONE WHO SAYS DIABETES IS A DISEASE THAT PEOPLE SHOULD JUST BE ABLE TO CONTROL EASILY: "I hear you. But you have to understand that diabetes looks one way on paper and entirely another in real life. Not making insulin? Take insulin. But with that request comes the real risk and accompanying real fear of low blood sugars that could cause seizures, coma, or death. It's a balance between taking too much insulin and not enough insulin, and a miscalculation is easy with so many shifting variables." *Insert awkward laugh.* "We make it look too easy at times, but it's not easy."

DESCRIBING TO SOMEONE WHO I HOPE WILL DONATE TO SUPPORT A DIABETES ORG: "I think about diabetes every night before I fall asleep. Because I'm never sure I'll wake up in the morning. When I'm alone at night with my kids, I wonder who will get them breakfast if I die while I'm sleeping. It sounds dramatic because it is a realistic worry. I never feel safe. I'm afraid that diabetes looks too easy or looks to manageable to folks on the outside, which might keep them from thinking it's serious. But it's deadly serious. We deserve funding for research and a cure. Until we're cured, every day we manage a serious amount of risk."

DESCRIBING TO MY CHILDREN: "Yes, I had a low blood sugar, but you know what? That's why I wear my Dexcom. And why we keep juice on that table. Mommy is always as careful and as prepared as possible. Because what's my job?" Long pause. "That's right, to take good care of you." Long hug. "I love you guys."

Cleaning Crews

The urge to clean grabs me by the throat, and I find myself spritzing Clorox on the counter and rubbing frantically with a fistful of paper towels. Once that task is accomplished, I notice that the floor just below the refrigerator door is sticky with juice or something, so I kneel down and scrub that, too. And then suddenly the fridge door needs a scrub down, and I should probably grab all the sweet potatoes that are growing actual faces there on the back shelf and I think there's a jar of minced garlic that's spilled somewhere in there and …

… all while the Dexcom wails, shouting "LOW!! KERRI!! STOP FRIGGING CLEANING AND EAT SOMETHING!!!"

I look at the graph and see the double-down arrows, and confirm the low with my meter. But it takes an awful lot of self-control to stop scrubbing and drink some grape juice.

Why am I struck with that urge to clean when I'm low? I do not understand what it is about the Low Cleaning Crew that moves into my brain when the sugar apparently moves out, but they are a merry and maniacal mix of maids.

When my blood sugar is in the absolute trenches, I get these cleaning fits. Emptying the dishwasher, folding laundry, picking up the piles of kid toys that little the floor … it's like the slow ebbing of glucose from my blood stream makes my body feel so disorganized and rattled that I search and destroy all external messes to level the proverbial playing field.

Usually, it's the beading of sweat on my forehead that makes me stop cleaning and acknowledge my blood sugar. A lot of times, that cleaning fit comes with a frantically panicked mindset, where my brain is racing to think as many thoughts in as little time as possible, my hands shaking open a new garbage bag or sliding forks and knives into their places in the drawer organizer.

"Did you have a low?" Chris asks, looking at the gleaming kitchen and the piles of folded clothes.

"How could you tell?" I responded, wiping the glucose dust off the kitchen counter with a swipe of my sleeve.

"Wild guess."

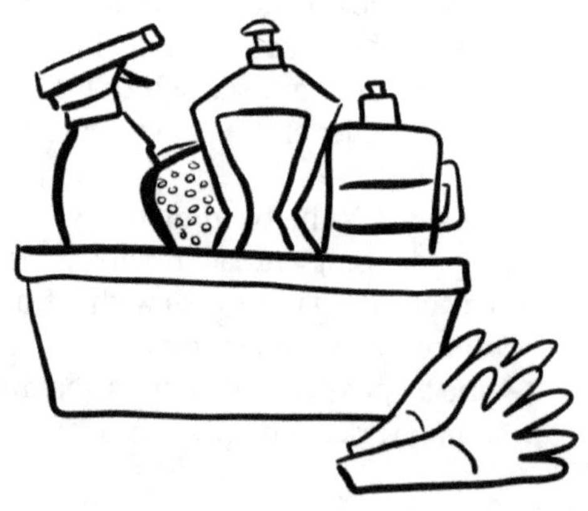

A Sobering Experience

"Do you mind ringing out this orange juice first?" I asked the lady who was working the cash register.

"No problem," and she went *bip* with the scanner against the bottle's bar code while my Dexcom screamed BEEP BEEP BEEP! from my phone.

I opened the bottle and downed the majority of it in one, open-throated gulp. My son, strapped into the front of the shopping cart, reached over to the conveyor belt as the groceries were unloaded, one by one, by his mother with the shaking hands.

"Hang on, little guy. Here, play with this," I said, handing him a crinkly toy elephant that was peeking out of my purse. I ran my sleeve against my forehead to catch the beads of sweat that threatened to run down my face. My ankles felt weak while I clumsily unloaded the contents of my carriage onto the conveyor belt.

"Miss, do you have a Stop & Shop card?" the cashier asked, surveying the scene playing out in front of her. She was my mother's age. She watched me fumble with my wallet in search of the card, and I dropped it instead of landing it into her hand.

"Hang on a second," I said, carefully bending over and plucking the card from the floor. My son yelled, "YEAH!!!" and then "HEY!" from the carriage. My blood sugar was still dropping and the Dexcom kept hollering. Clumsy hands and the fog of hypoglycemia made my every movement look ridiculously awkward.

And I knew, knew, knew that the cashier thought I was drunk.

Hypoglycemic episodes can look like drunk moments, but I hadn't ever been mistaken as drunk when low before. In college, I had this credit-card sized placard in my wallet that said something like, "I have type 1 diabetes. If I seem drunk, please allow me to check my blood sugar to make sure I am not experiencing low blood sugar." I never had to use it, and my college roommates and I giggled at it once in a while, probably because we were actually drunk.

But yesterday at the grocery store, I wished that card had been in my wallet. I would have handed it to the cashier and pointed sheepishly at the orange juice.

Instead, in the fog of my low, I gracelessly unloaded and paid for my groceries while wrangling my one-year-old. Running my debit card for the purchase, I said to the cashier, "I have diabetes. My blood sugar is low," but I'm not sure she believed me. My brain wasn't sweetened enough to care. I was more concerned with pushing through to the other side of this low.

After we paid, I moved the carriage over to a row of benches just inside the main door of the grocery store and we sat there. I finished my orange juice. A few minutes later, the arrow on my CGM graph started pointing in a more respectable direction. I almost went back to the cashier to explain myself more lucidly but decided against it. Maybe next time I see her, I'll explain. For now, it was time to go home.

"Mama? Mamamamamamamama …" rambled my little man.

"Okay, sweet boy. We're good to go. Let's go."

Evidence

I opened my eyes slowly, taking a second at least to convince my lids to lift.

Oh, home. I'm in my own bed.

Moved my hand towards the cellphone on my bedside table, in pursuit of my continuous glucose monitor graph. My hand moved in slow motion, a trace of its movement in the air behind it.

53 mg/dL.

"Not that low, but low enough," my brain acknowledged, and my head went to nod but its response time was dulled. The connection between "do this action" and "this action" was entirely severed. My body didn't want to do anything unless it was to have my hands twitch mildly and my eyelids to shut.

A juice box sat, untouched, on the bedside table. It's right there. Right there. I'm still here, still here, not reaching for it.

My brain is displeased, logical and panicking and screaming.

GET THE GODDAMN JUICE AND DRINK IT WHAT ARE YOU WAITING FOR YOU ARE FALLING DOWN THIS WELL OF HYPOGLYCEMIA. DO SOMETHING BEFORE YOU DROWN. GET UP GET UP. GET UP.

Sure, brain. I'll grab that juice box.

… in a minute.

It's not like falling down a well with gravity providing an assist; it's going down the shaft of a well like Alice falling into Wonderland, floaty and confusing and hard to make my body respond to the commands of my brain. I would have closed my eyes tight in order to concentrate on actions but they wouldn't close tight. They only wanted to stare at the ceiling for a few seconds before fluttering shut again.

A minute or thirty passed and it seemed that I had drank the juice box. The empty box with the straw poking out as evidence. The stain of grape juice on my sheets - evidence. My hands and eyes and legs doing what I requested, more evidence.

Still here. Evidence.

Swing over to the side of the bed. I sent the message to my legs. They responded gratefully and almost instantly, coming out from underneath the thick winter blankets, my feet touching the floor for the first time of this earned day. Stretched my arms over my head, wobbly and still not back in range yet but I'm still here. Still here.

Still here.

Good Luck, Lady

I went to my dentist appointment.

"Aaaaaaaaahhhhh," I opened my mouth like a baby bird every time the hygienist came near me. I couldn't answer any of her questions because my toes were curling with fear. Those metal instruments scraping against my sensitive teeth and poking mercilessly at my gums.

"Aaaaaaaahhhhh!" as I caught my reflection in the mirror as the blood was seeping out from around my gums. Panic struck me. I tried to stay calm, reaching down oh so slowly to put the pump on "Suspend" mode, as my nerves make my blood sugar plummet. "You okay?" the hygienist asked, scraping across my molar and making the hair on my arms shudder.

"I'm fine. Just keep going." I said, only though a mouth full of her fingers. So it sounded more like "Ib fibe. Tuskeeb go en."

She finished me up. I escaped the office, nerves on edge but satisfied that I was safe for another six months. I put the key into the ignition of the car, pushed aside the dangling tendrils of the hibiscus plant (I'll explain in a minute), and headed towards what was scheduled to become my new home.

My car was teeming with the last minute items from the move. In making sure my old apartment was completely empty, I had to forgo the rational "packing" course and opt for "tossing things haphazardly into the car" mode. A bag full of cleaning supplies, a roll of paper towels, and my snow boots rustled about on the back seat. An African Violet teetered precariously on the floor. And my giant hibiscus plant was everywhere. Long branches with big pink flowers were bobbing up and down every time I accelerated too aggressively.

I advanced up the road. Not feeling too great, but I had just come from the Evil Dentist's Office so I chalked up my headache to that.

I was on the phone with Chris as I drove, but realized that I felt bizarre.

"I am going to pull over. I think I need to test." I told him. He urged me to do just that. "I'll wait on the phone with you," he said.

Pulled over. Grabbed the meter. The lancet hit my fingertip. The blood drop, then the countdown.

5...4...3...2...1 ... **40 mg/dl.**

"Holy shit, Chris. I'm 40. I need to get some juice or something."

He remained on the phone as I pulled into the nearby gas station. "Get some juice." "Okay, okay." I told him I would call him right back, as soon as I bought and drank some juice.

I stumbled into the gas station, lost in my own head. Headache: check. Dizzy: check. Arms and legs weak, as though they'd run a marathon the rest of me didn't attend: check. But my mind was frighteningly clear. I knew exactly what was going on. I knew I needed to make it to the back of the store, where the coolers were, grab a juice and throw it down as fast as possible.

These waves of nausea and dizziness swept over me. I felt them starting in my ankles, rising up to my waist and cresting just over my eyes, rendering me lost for a second. I paused in walking while the waves washed over me. And I held out my hands to brace myself if I fell as I made my way towards the coolers.

Sometimes a low blood sugar just wrecks you thoroughly.

Grabbed the cold glass doors and swung them open. Dole Orange Juice ... the bottle looked so familiar, like I'd been dreaming about it. In one motion, I uncapped the bottle, drank the juice, and eased my shaking frame against the doors.

The man behind the counter didn't see me struggling at the back of his store. He didn't notice that tears were running down my face as I brought the empty juice bottle to his register to pay for it. The cell phone, open and dialed to Chris's number, was hanging limply from my hands.

"You want pay for that bottle?"

"Yes. Please. My name is Kerri." I didn't want to tell him my name but I couldn't help but think that if he knew my name then I would be safer.

"One dollar. Forty-nine cents. You want a ticket?"

"Yes. Please. I'm having a diabetic low blood sugar reaction." I offered a weak smile, handing him my money.

"Juice. Tickets. Here. Good luck, lady."

Keys in the ignition, I tried to relax as the sugar eased into my blood stream. I called Chris and promptly started to cry at his "Are you okay? Did you drink the juice?"

"I'm fine. I drank the juice. I'll be okay..." The plastic bag rustled as I threw in the empty bottle of juice. The arms of the giant hibiscus flowers eased around my shoulders.

It wasn't until I was driving back home, blood sugar stabilized at 97 mg/dl, that I realized there were two lottery tickets clutched in my hand.

Low Hangovers

The alarm went off. I couldn't shake the sleep from my body.

This morning, I swept the empty carcasses of two juice boxes off the bedside table, a reminder of what must have happened last night. I looked at my CGM graph and saw a line with the shape of a teaspoon etched into it around 2.30 am, where I spent 45 minutes alarming in response to the LOW.

"Huh," I said, running my hands along the fitted sheet as I made the bed, seeing the small blot of grape juice on the edge of the fabric. My body felt chilled, a reminder that the overnight hypo caused me to sweat through my pajamas, leaving me still slightly damp around my shoulders, hair frizzy-curled at the ends. "Need to run these sheets through the wash today."

Everything felt a little heavier, a little slower, on a half second delay that wasn't enough for anyone else to notice but more than enough for me to go downstairs with a hand firmly on the railing. Low hangovers require more recovery time, these days. They linger.

I have no recollection of last night's low blood sugar. An hour of activity, but I don't remember it. No memory of popping the straw through the foil hole of the juice box, twice over. No memory of the Dexcom alarm going off, although I have evidence on my phone that it alarmed several times. No memory of waking up damp with sweat and nerves.

The only proof of hypoglycemia is in the trash can, on the sheets, pressed into my graph, and under my eyes.

Parking Lot Lows

"Brrrrr ... it's a little chilly outside today," I said to BSparl as I tucked her blanket snug around her wiggly little self in the car seat. She waved at me and showed me her sock.

"Yes, that's a nice sock, birdy. Okay, let's get out of here and get you into the car so we can go home!"

The automatic doors parted and a brisk gust of wind came and skipped down my collar.

With the baby's car seat safely tucked into the belly of the carriage, I ventured out to find my car in the massive parking lot.

"Ha ha, where did Mommy leave the car?" I said out loud, walking up and down the parking lot aisles and pressing the alarm on my keys. Nothing. No flashing lights, no subtle little "beep" noise from my Honda. Nothing but a sea of cars and I had no idea which one was mine.

"Am I getting old?" I asked BSparl.

"Mmmmmm!" she proclaimed, raising her teething toy into the air.

I walked for several minutes, combing the lot for my car. And the wind kept whipping, only this time it felt good because it kept whisking the sweat off the nape of my neck. I felt dizzy.

"This car has to be here somewhere ..." I passed the same minivan I had just seen moments ago, the one with the stickers on the back of a stick figure family. "I just can't find it. I can't find anything, baby. I have no idea where this car is."

BSparl was starting to fall asleep, tucked happily into the blankets in her car seat. And I could not find the car. The parking lot was this sea of blue and black and red cars, none of which were mine. My vision began to sharpen on the peripheral, leaving my main point of focus a little blurrier than usual. The sounds of the parking lot were magnified in my head, leaving me confused and lost in my mental cotton ball.

I felt the buzzing from my purse, and then heard the unmistakable BEEEEEEEP! of the Dexcom. Without checking to see what my blood sugar was, I reached into my purse while pushing the carriage and retrieved a jar of glucose tabs. I chomped down on four of them at a time, the glucose dust taking off into the air.

The ground was starting to shift, like a blurry and constant tremor that only I felt. I knew this low wasn't good - I needed to find my car and sit in a hurry. But I had the baby with me. I had to make sure she was safe, too.

I saw a young kid who was corralling the shopping carts. I motioned for him to come over, and he trotted over with a half-smile.

"You okay?" he asked.

"Not really. I'm having a low blood sugar reaction and I cannot find my car. I need to get my baby into the car and out of the cold, but I can't find my car. It's not here. I can't find it." I hate when crying is the prominent symptom of a low. I felt the tears coming. And then I started to laugh, because I was picturing myself, shopping cart crammed with baby and bags, my coat sleeves covered in glucose dust, crying and roaming aimlessly around the parking lot in search of one little car.

This poor kid must have thought I was on drugs.

Everything happened in fast forward. This kid told me to stay where I was and he would find my car. He took my keys and returned quickly, telling me I was just a few aisles over. He put the baby's car seat in her car, loaded my bags into my trunk, and asked me if I was okay. I inhaled a few more glucose tabs in the meantime.

"Do you need me to call someone for you?"

"No, I'll be fine in just a few minutes. I just couldn't find the stupid car and my blood sugar wasn't helping. I'm so sorry. Thank you so much for your help."

"Okay. No problem. If you need anything, I'll be rounding up carts. I will be watching you, okay?" He paused for a second, and then rubbed his hands over his attempt at a beard. "Not like 'watching you' in a creepy way. Just like making sure you two are okay."

I sat in the car and waited for my blood sugar to come up while BSparl napped in the back seat. After a few minutes, I checked to see 82 mg/dl flashing up from my meter.

"Holy biplane-building cats, Batman," I mumbled to myself. "I must have been crazy low."

Safe in my car with my baby buckled in, I waited in the parking lot for my blood sugar to continue to rise, thankful for the kindness of strangers.

Whine

I woke up high this morning, thanks to a late-night snack of quinoa that didn't get into my system fully until well after I'd gone to bed. Pre-bedtime test was 94 mg/dl, but I woke up at 7:30 am with a full bladder, sweaters on the ol' teeth, a backache, small ketones, and a blood sugar of 298 mg/dl. I cranked in a correction bolus and went about getting ready for work.

I don't usually fall fast after highs. It takes me about two hours to really settle back into a steadier range, and sometimes longer to even start the blood sugar tumble. I showered, reconnected the pump, got dressed in a hurry, and shuffled my almost-always-late ass out the door. Mind you, only 38 minutes had passed from the time I bolused.

Got to work, turned on my computer, and started picking through my work emails. But I had that feeling of foggy distraction - the sound of a coworker tapping her fingers against the keys were resonating in my brain too loudly. I clicked on "new" about three times before realizing that I was trying to "reply" to an email instead. Brain was malfunctioning. I tested my blood sugar, knowing something was up.

Or down, since the result was 53 mg/dl and falling fast.

I reached into my small, compact work bag (lie: the bag is enormous and I'll end up deformed from carrying around so much unnecessary crap) and pulled out a bottle of juice I'd had stashed for a few weeks. It was a bottle I used at the gym once before and just refilled for an emergency. I twisted off the cap and heard a distinct hiss, like I woke up an angry grape juice rattle snake.

Juice doesn't normally hiss, does it?

I gave the contents a quick sniff and realized that the grape juice had fermented and was now spoiled and closer to "wine" than "reaction treater." Thankfully, I had a can of juice in the fridge at work, so a quick pull helped elevate my blood sugar.

Kerri, take note (from yourself in third person): Juice becomes wine when you have it go from hot to cold a million times. No juice when you're low becomes whine. Though the pun is delightful, stick with glucose tabs, okay? They're less apt to spoil.

Hypo Effery

BEEEEEPBEEEEEPBEEEEEP!!

My purse start vibrating in a panic.

79 mg/dL and two arrows down – how the hell did that happen? I just dropped my daughter off at preschool. My blood sugar was 139 mg/dL before leaving the house with a steady, easterly arrow.

I pulled the car over and put on my hazard lights so I could bust out my glucose meter. (Hell yes I treat low blood sugars purely based on a Dexcom reading from a trusted sensor, but this sensor is on Day 14 and due to be changed this afternoon, so my trust was getting rusty. Trusty? Rustworthy. Bah.) Meter said 68 mg/dL.

The symptoms, which weren't strong when I pulled over, were starting to edge in. Shaky hands and blurred vision (almost wrote "blurred bison," which sounds like a band name) paved the way for clammy skin, which let the fog of hypoglycemia settle into my brain.

Fine then. I reached into the glove compartment for the ubiquitous jar of glucose tabs. Chomp, chomp on four of them only to realize they aren't Glucolift (there were so tasty – Google them) but instead the generic chalkified glucose tabs from CVS and became grossed out. The low symptoms were intensifying as I sat on the side of the road, so being picky about my glucose sources wasn't an option. Chomp, chomp on another tab, wishing I could somehow keep a soft-serve ice cream machine in the glove compartment instead.

Moments pass. I'm still buckled into my car, eating snacks, watching cars whiz by. The Dexcom finally shows an upward climbing arrow. My hairline feels less clammy. The shape of the steering wheel and the radio control knobs come back into sharp focus.

Better.

"Did you check your GPS?" my mom asks me whenever we're about to get into the car together.

"Mom, it's a CGM. And yes, I did check it," I reply, usually laughing because no matter how many times I tell her it's a CGM, she still calls it a GPS.

But as I think about what may have happened if the low symptoms hit in full while I was driving instead of after I had pulled over, GPS might me just as accurate, giving me the location, in context, of what the hell my blood sugars are doing.

Pulled Over

I had just buckled the girls into their car seats and was ready to make the drive home from day camp, and as I turned the car on, I reflexively grabbed my Dexcom receiver to take a peek at my blood sugars before I started driving.

Shit. 68 mg/dL with an arrow straight down and a blood drop signaling a need for calibration.

"Hang on guys," I said to my daughter and her friend, who were already singing camp songs in the backseat. "I need to wait a minute before we head out." I pricked my finger quickly to check my blood sugar and, sure enough, saw the 63 mg/dL on my meter waving its arms at me. No worries – I always have a jar of glucose tabs in my center console.

Except this time.

Shit.

"Hey girls. Do you guys have anything left in your lunches?"

"Yeah, I have strawberries and a pouch left in my lunch. Do you want it, Mom?" Birdy offered.

"Yep." I climbed out of the car and went back to the trunk to rummage around through her lunch bag. Pulling out the snacks, I gobbled them while standing at the back of my car, a mom on a mission to bring her blood sugar up before driving.

We sat in the parking lot for ten minutes or so, and I watched the CGM graph arrow relax and point sideways. A glucose meter check showed me at 78 mg/dL, so I felt I was on the rise. We started the ride home.

Except the CGM alarm went off 15 minutes later, only this time it showed double-down arrows and the BELOW 55 mg/dL message on the screen.

"Shit."

Certain parts of Rhode Island are relatively rural, and sometimes you have to drive for a while before you pass a gas station or a convenience store. I immediately started calculating when I'd pass the next place to stop. I also assessed my symptoms (none) and instinctively reached over to disconnect my insulin pump from my hip. I thought the two little kids in my car. I thought about where I could pull over. I worried about what was safer: driving for another minute or pulling over and not having any food in the car. And I hoped that worrying so intensely would make me feel stressed and hopefully jack my blood sugar up a little more. (Come on, cortisol!)

Just ahead, I saw the familiar orange and brown sign of a Dunkin' Donuts coffee shop.

"Yes." I put on my blinker and pulled into the drive through lane of the coffee shop. "Girls, I need to stop here and get an orange juice, okay?"

"DOUGHNUTS!!!!!" they yelled in unison.

"Not this time, guys. I need to get some juice and wait a few more minutes before we can keep going."

Minutes later, I was in the parking lot with an empty bottle of orange juice and two kids in the backseat of the car who were peppering me with questions about diabetes.

"Why did we have to stop?"

"Because I needed juice to treat a low blood sugar."

"What's a low blood sugar," asked my daughter's friend.

Birdy piped up. "It's when you have diabetes and you have too much insulin or not enough food in your body and you need glucose tabs or juice or doughnuts but not today." (All in one breath.)

"No doughnuts?"

"Sorry, guys."

"Can we drive soon?"

"Yes."

"Okay, can we sing until we start driving?"

"Sure."

We sat in the parking lot while I waited for the orange juice to do its thing, keeping an eye on my CGM graph and an ear on the two little kids in the back of my car who were belting out songs they learned at camp and who trusted me to take good care of myself in order to take good care of them.

Only no doughnuts.

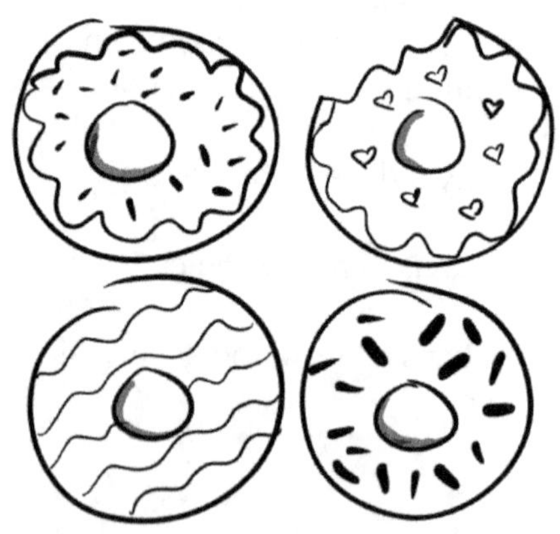

Half a Juice Box

Turn on the light.

Fall back asleep.

Press the button on the CGM to make it stop beeping.

Fall back asleep.

Unzip the meter case and take out my glucose meter.

Lapse back into sleep again; was it sleep or was I passed out and what's the difference when it's 4 am and your blood sugar is under 40 mg/dL?

Opting for a juice box instead of the open jar of glucose tabs on my bedside table, I fumbled with the straw and once it hit the foil-covered mark, I drank as though my life depended on it.

Because it felt, in that moment, like it did.

I was 98% sure I would be completely fine in a few minutes, with no lasting effect of the severe low except maybe a hypoglycemia hangover. But until the juice hit my system and my brain stopped panicking, the 2% of doubt invaded every bit of me.

"I wasn't afraid I was going to die," I told Chris, explaining the next morning why I was so tired. "It was more like I was really aware of how close I was to a dangerous physical state, and I needed to make sure I didn't cross the threshold, whatever that might be."

"I wish I had heard the alarm. We need to do something about that – you need to keep it in a glass even when I'm home, so I can hear it when you don't. I need to be able to hear it, too," he said, giving my shoulders a squeeze.

"Yeah, but what's weird is that all I could think about, as I was waiting to come up and feeling pretty awful, I kept debating whether or not to drink the rest of the juice box instead of just drinking half. I wanted to drink the whole thing, and then fifteen other juice boxes and maybe a sandwich, for good measure. But instead, I was sweating and shaking and confused and at the bottom of the well, you know? And the only moment of clarity I had was limiting myself to half of a juice box, knowing it would bring me up just enough and not too much."

Having the first half saves my life, and having the wherewithal to not drink the second half saves me high blood sugars when I wake up. It's humbling, realizing what hangs in the balance of half a juice box.

Oh, High!

Sunday morning started off with promise - a fasting blood sugar of 99 mg/dL, a healthy breakfast of tea, a banana, and some scrambled eggs, and I remembered to grab my curling iron out of the fridge before meeting my ride to the airport.

I took an aggressive bolus for breakfast (because travel sometimes makes me run a bit higher, for a multitude of reasons), so I was surprised to see double-up arrows on my Dexcom graph while I was standing in the airport security line.

"Hmmm ... 172 and double ups ... with three units of insulin on board." The diabetes mental-math made sense to me. "I'm going to let this blood sugar ride out instead of rage blousing."

But by the time I was in my seat on the plane, I was at 312 mg/dL. I do not know why. I calculated breakfast. I bolused well before I ate. And I didn't feel stressed or nervous or whatever.

But now I was high. And I felt high. High, high, high.

It's a thick feeling in the base of your brain, like someone's cracked open your head and replaced your gray matter with sticky jam. I find myself zoning out and staring at things, and my eyeballs feel dry and like they're tethered to my head by frayed ropes instead of optic nerves. Everything is slow and heavy and whipped with heavy cream.

During the first hour of my flight from Austin to Baltimore, I tried to write but the words were stuck in my teeth. I tried to read a book but I kept skimming the same sentences over and over again without really reading them. And I watched my blood sugar holding steady in the 300's, despite my boluses.

Rage bolusing is a hard thing for me to avoid, especially once I'm so deep into a high blood sugar that I'd do just about anything for a bottle of water and a 120 mg/dL.

When I'm high, my back aches. My eyes hurt. My breath smells like the glue you use to assemble model airplanes. My whole body is wrapped in cotton balls and I'm reduced to a lazy, lethargic lump in a seat, without a shred of energy and zero desire to smile. I want to bang on the buttons of my pump, ringing through a billion units. I want to know why my breakfast bolus didn't make a dent, and why these subsequent "fix it" boluses aren't doing shit. Is my infusion set crapped out? Is my insulin vial spoiled? Am I dehydrated? Did I miscalculate my breakfast bolus? Did one of the fifteen thousand diabetes variables go rogue on me?

I didn't want to swap out my infusion set in the bathroom on the plane and then have to wait, wait, impatiently wait to see if another bolus will hit my bloodstream. I tested my blood sugar again and saw that I was up to 360 mg/dL, and the Dexcom graph didn't show any promise of a drop anytime soon.

Which is how I ended up busting out my insulin pen on the flight, about two hours into my flight, sneaking in a quick injection into my belly while the girl next to me read her biology textbook. (She didn't notice. Even after all these years on a pump, I can still manage to inject discreetly.)

By the time I was on my connection flight, I had settled back into a less rage-ish range. Was it the string of small boluses, finally catching up with me? Can I thank the injection? Either way, the molasses in my veins had been replaced, once more, by blood. Game over for diabetes chaos.

And looking at my Dexcom graph, I realize that diabetes gives a whole new meaning to "mile high club."

Pregnancy and Parenting

Pregnancy and Parenting

If there was an ability to fast-forward through the whole pregnancy bit and get to the baby-in-your-arms moment, that would have been terrific. The pressure and panic of growing a child in my own body was intense; medical professionals had always discussed pregnancy as a "hmmm, maybe," there weren't a lot of examples of a healthy pregnancy with diabetes for me to reference, and I was not confident that a body which had failed me a few times was going to deliver on the baby-making details.

On my website, I wrote long, detailed posts about my pregnancies. Some of the stuff would feel familiar to most (adjusting to a growing body, the weird pregnancy quicks of swollen ankles and emotions swirling on spin cycle, etc). A lot of the other stuff was about diabetes specifically, like how my insulin needs changed throughout a pregnancy, or how breastfeeding affected my blood sugars. Part of my experience included infertility and pregnancy loss, and while those essays are not specifically included here, they are very much a part of my journey to becoming a parent. The diabetes nitty-gritty was also important to me in terms of telling my story, because it was the stuff I wondered most about when I was considering pregnancy. Did I overshare? Hell yes, I believe I did.

The essays included in this section focus on how diabetes influences my parenting. About how we include diabetes into our conversations, and how we inform our children about this chronic illness. About how diabetes explains some of what we do and how we plan, but it doesn't keep us from creating families and loving them intensely.

Moody, Pregnant Mess

This is one of those essays I'll write, and then promptly wish I hadn't written, but then revisit in a few weeks and be thankful that I let these emotions out. But for now, I want to hide in bed and stay there all day, even though I can't sleep because my guilt is keeping me awake.

I am not sure what's causing what, but my emotions feel like they're in a tailspin today. Over Friday and Saturday, I had blood sugars that seemed like they came straight from the store - shiny, flat, and steady, with the Dexcom showing me a straight line for over 24 hours (aside from one very small spike after pineapple and cottage cheese on Saturday morning) and with the meter confirming this anomaly every hour or so. And BSparl was poking and kicking around in there, letting me know that she was alive and okay and having a good time floating in her safe, amniotic sea.

And then, for absolutely no reason, I had two rotten lows in a three hour span. Rotten as in sweaty, dizzy, Dexcom wailing at me, orange juice spilled on the kitchen floor due to downing it too quickly from the carton kind of lows. Lows that left me needing a nap and feeling physically compromised.

And I worried about her - this little friend I'm building.

Of course, these lows were followed by highs. Tricky highs - ones that made my mouth dry and my head hurt and my blood sugar average leap up by at least 20 points all on their own. Highs that made me test, bolus, and then go into the bathroom and cry because I felt so guilty about what I was doing to myself and to this little kid. (Granted, the crying part may have happened because of the hormone influx, but I can't tell what's causing what these days.)

I have these books that I bought after finding out about BSparl - volumes with titles like "What to Expect When You're Expecting" and "I'm Pregnant!" - and for weeks, I pored through them and read all about how the baby was growing from a little cluster of cells into a creature with arms and legs and a beating heart. But these books all come with what I call the "scary chapters," about complications and all the crap that can go wrong during pregnancy. I skimmed these chapters at the outset, felt completely overwhelmed and terrified, and decided to not read them anymore. Then we had the scare with the bleeding back in September (where I was about 7 weeks along and there were no problems detected, but my heart remained in my throat for ... actually, not sure if it's come down at all yet), and I decided that I wanted to stick my head in the sand and pretend that nothing bad is even possible. Every pregnant woman has a healthy, happy pregnancy, and that's it. That's the only route, right?

I know that diabetics have healthy babies all the time. And that in the grand scheme of things, it's not about each individual blood sugar, but the general gist of how my blood sugars are running. But I've only read about other people's pregnancies. I've never been pregnant before, and all of these feelings, both physically and emotionally, are so new to me. Even though there are so many examples of families before me who have taken this journey and come out safely and happy on the other side, I've never done it before. I don't know what I'm doing. I'm scared a lot of the time because I don't want to hurt her.

This morning, after going to bed at a blood sugar of 119 mg/dl, I woke up around 5:45 am at 293 mg/dl. I took a correction bolus, tested for ketones (none), drank a bottle of water to hydrate my sandpaper throat, and then climbed back into bed.

(Mind you, this high was on the same basal rates that have had me waking up under 100 mg/dl for three days running.)

And couldn't sleep.

My mind keeps freaking out, going back to the scary chapters. And no amount of rationalization (it's just a few hours high, it's just one blood sugar, it's just one bad day, everyone has those bad days, the baby is okay, you're okay) could make my mind quiet. I just feel like a failure, frustrated to tears because no matter how much technology we have access to as modern-day diabetics, we still have diabetes. And this obscene disease looks so quiet from the outside, but it rages on inside of me every day, even when I'm working so hard to pretend to be cured for my daughter.

It's going to be better. Now that I've finished this post, my number is back down to 131 mg/dl and falling slowly, and within the next 20 minutes or so, I'll be back in range. And I'm hoping that I can stay on top of things today and keep her safe.

Six months pregnant tomorrow.

I've never wanted anything more than this, in my entire life. I might sound overly dramatic or obsessive or frantic, but I can't lie. This baby girl is so important to me, and she may be the only child we have. She's what I've been thinking about for years, and she just rolled inside of me right now, as if to say, "It's cool, mommy. Stop freaking out. Let's have pancakes!"

I should make her some pancakes.

I feel better now. It feels good to get these thoughts out of my head for a bit. Thank you for listening.

Ignoring Her

She was tucked into the bassinet, perfectly safe and sound. Only she was wailing, with this loud cry and her bottom lip pouted out at an impossible angle, because she was hungry.

"I'm sorry, baby girl. You have to wait just a few minutes so Mommy can have some juice, okay?"

I was standing at her side, belly full of grape juice and a blood sugar of 43 mg/dl.

BSparl needed to eat, I needed to breastfeed her, but I didn't feel confident picking her up just yet. Of course, she started to cry just as the meter tossed that result at me. A perfect storm of chaos. My hands were too shaky and my brain wasn't 100% tuned in to reality. She was safe and unharmed, but her cries were cutting through me and settling right in like barbed wire around my heart.

"Two more minutes, sweetie. Can you hang on?" I stood by the bassinet and stroked her hair while she cried.

"Why, Mom? Why aren't you picking me up and feeding me? You're right there! I can see you! I can smell you! I hear your voice! Why? Mommy, pick me uuuuuuuup!"

(Or at least that's what I heard in her cries. I'm sure it was some variation on that theme.)

Within a few more minutes, I felt much better. More capable of picking up my daughter and bringing her over to the couch so I could feed her. I kept a jar of glucose tabs on the coffee table while I fed BSparl, and the Dexcom eventually showed some arrows pointing north (it was like a CGM "thumbs up"). And we were both fine. BSparl ate, I was fine, and we moved on with our day.

But the guilt of not giving her what she needs is something I need to adjust to. In keeping with the idea of making sure my proverbial oxygen mask is on before assisting my child, I need to be in good form in order to take good care of my kid. That means that my blood sugar needs to come first. And that also means that my kid has to fuss while I wait for my blood sugar to be at a more reasonable level. I can't pick her up if I feel shaky. And I can't let the sound of her cries make me make decisions that aren't safe.

... it's hard, though! Her bottom lip is ENORMOUS, and it's like my body is programmed to respond when she cries. Leaving her there in the bassinet while I went to drink juice was heartbreaking, because she doesn't understand why I'm not giving her what she needs. I don't want her to think her mommy is ignoring her. The time will come when she understands how this balance works. She'll grow up knowing that food is sometimes medicine and that her mommy, though madly in love with her, can't do it all at once.

Until then, I'll stand at the bassinet and stroke her head, hoping that she'll why I let her cry.

Things I Learned in my First Year as a Mom with Diabetes

Things I learned during my first year as a mom with diabetes:

- Not all women with diabetes have c-sections. I did, but it doesn't make me the rule. C-section deliveries are the exception.
- A pregnancy with diabetes, even well-controlled diabetes, can have its share of complications. This does not mean I failed.
- I quickly learned to stash fruit roll ups in the couch cushions for breastfeeding lows.
- Writing my blood sugar level on the bags of pumped breast milk helped instill the confidence that my blood sugar level didn't affect the quality of my milk.
- Carrying the car seat against my hip can accidentally bolus my pump.
- So can sticky little baby fingers.
- When she has to wait while I treat a low blood sugar, it makes me hate diabetes so intensely that my eyebrows hurt from furrowing them.
- Test strips on the floor aren't a big deal until she tries to eat them.
- Bottles of glucose tabs make for the best impromptu rattles.
- I didn't realize she was able to pull my pump from my hip and crawl off with it until I felt the site pull loose.
- Between the baby bag, the diabetes supplies, and "regular life" stuff, I am bound to leave something behind. But so long as that "something" isn't me or her, we're fine.
- While I don't always know the lyrics, I do know the tune. And I'm like the Wayne Brady of makeshift mommy lyrics.
- I've never, in my life, had such in-depth discussions about poop and blood sugar numbers, all in the same breath. ("Dude, she's taking a massive crap right now, but I'm 50 and I need to grab some juice. Can you take this hit?")
- Going to the beach is hard when you bring two kids under six months of age. (It gets easier. RIGHT? Please God.)

- I wasn't prepared for how sad I would be to pack up her too-small clothes, but I felt so proud to buy her first sippy cup.
- I've never ordered so much crap online in such a short span.
- Going gluten-free for the first year was doable enough to encourage us to maybe aim for a few more months.
- And in the last twelve months, I've learned to be very comfortable, and unflappable, about my decisions on how to parent my child.
- When she slept through the night and her diaper was soggy, I thought, "She slept through the night!" and not "Does she have diabetes?"
- Gluten-free crackers taste nice. Gluten-free pasta is not so nice.
- Nothing entertains her more than my Dexcom receiver. She likes the beeps, the lights, and the plastic gel case. It is the ultimate tantrum deterrent.
- Baby Mum Mums are delicious. There. I said it.
- Working from home gave me the privilege and pleasure of not missing a moment of my baby's first year, time to safely manage new motherhood and diabetes, and instilled a true appreciation for "time to myself."
- After twelve months, the laundry is still adorable but the diapers are less so. (Nothing to do with diabetes. But her clothes are cute overload in the dryer.)
- Being her mom makes me want to have the nicest A1C ever, so I can be around to bug her for a long, long time.

My first year as a mom has taught me a tremendous amount - more than one essay could ever cover - and I learn more about my kid (and my marriage and myself and spit up and toys that require 15 batteries and have a cleverly-hidden off switch) every day.

This is what I've learned. BUT. I've yet to learn how to install the car seat base on my own. Which makes Chris my hero forever.

How I Talk about Diabetes to my Kids

During a conference discussion about being a parent with type 1 diabetes, the topic of "telling" came up over and over again. And not "telling" as in "I'm telling on you, pancreas, for being a lazy slab of cellular mass," but more how to tell my daughter about diabetes.

The people in the session had varying opinions, ranging from having a sit-down discussion about what the impact of diabetes may or may not be to introducing diabetes on a bit-by-bit basis, and all the gray area in between.

I definitely fall into that second camp, as a parent. My daughter is two years old. I don't want to have a formal sit-down chat with her about her mommy's diabetes, because it won't matter a lick to her unless it involves Thomas the Tank Engine or watering the flowers outside and she has absolutely no concept of what "chronic illness" means.

She's two.

However, like most kids, she's perceptive. She's been watching me test my blood sugar since she was able to hold her head up, and she has a sense of what it means to "check my finger" because she's also had her blood sugar checked a handful of times. She knows it's not a fun moment. ("That's mama's meh-cine. Not mines. You keep it.")

Lately, she's been asking to see the numbers as they count down. "Five, mama! Four! Three! Two! One!" And when the blood sugar number pops up, she reads that back to me. "Two eight, mama!" At which point I correct her: "No, you're reading it backwards. Eight two. Eighty-two." "Eighty-two! That's nice."

(Every number is "that's nice." 212 mg/dL? "That's nice." 182? 103? Eleven million and seven? "That's nice." I like that she thinks they're all nice. Makes me less bananas about them.)

"Twelve! You has a twelve, mama!! That's nice." She looks at my meter and announces the result proudly.

"One hundred and twelve, kiddo. But it is nice!"

She is learning about how the Dexcom receiver and the sensor on my thigh work together, especially now that it's summer and my sensor sometimes peeks out from underneath my shorts or dresses. "That's Dexcom." She picks up the Dexcom receiver. "That's Dexcom, too. Two Dexcoms!" Pause. "Ah, ah, ah!!" (We watch a fair amount of Sesame Street, and The Count is a fan favorite.) But last week, when the Dexcom alarmed for a blood sugar over 160 mg/dL, she grabbed the receiver off the kitchen table and said, "Mama, time for check your meh-cine!" The beeps mean something to her.

"Diabeeeeeeeetes." She knows the word. She knows that all of my medicine bits (the pump, the infusion set, the Dexcom, the sensor, the glucose meter, the glucose tabs ... all the "stuff") are related to this thing we keep calling "diabetes." She has no idea what it really means (pancreas kaput, etc.), but she is beginning to understand that it makes me do things differently than some of the other mommies.

My little Bird will make sense of my diabetes breadcrumb by breadcrumb, learning from the information I share with her. Eventually, as she grows older, we'll gently teach her what to do if Mommy needs help. She'll understand that I wear certain devices and take medicine before I eat and I sometimes wait a few extra minutes before we play outside, waiting for my blood sugar to come up. She'll know what she needs to know, but I don't want her to know any more than she needs to know. The parts of diabetes that scare me will be shielded from her for as long as I can, because there's no reason to make her worry.

My job is to love her. To play with her. For my husband and I to raise her as best we can, so that she becomes the best she can. My diabetes may impact certain moments, but it doesn't change the course of she is. Or who she will become.

Iron Mom

"I really like Iron Man. And Superman. And Spiderman." She paused. "But not the Hulk, because he smashes things. Why he smashes things?"

"He gets angry and that anger makes him turn into the giant green guy, and he smashes."

My daughter, thanks to her father's affinity for all-things superhero, has developed a taste for the slate of superheroes and super villains. She rocks her Superman t-shirt at school, and her Batman pajamas at home with both encouraging regularity and vigor. But that's the nature of her being three years old – she is learning so much every day, taking in her surroundings and chewing on them until they make sense for her.

Part of what she's hyper-fixated on, in addition to superheroes, is the location of my Dexcom and insulin pump. At least once a day, she asks me to show her my devices.

"Where is your Dexcom, mawm?" she asks me, patting my leg knowingly.

"Right here, on my right leg."

"And your pump is right here, right?" she asks, pressing her finger against the screen.

"Exactly."

The other day, Birdy was troubled because she couldn't find my insulin pump in the dress I was wearing. "Mom, where is your pump?"

"It's in the front of my dress, here," I said, pointing to where the pump was clipped to my bra, the screen facing out.

She contemplated this for a minute, and I could see the list of information she's been collecting in the last few weeks rolling around in the dryer of her mind.

"You're like Iron Man, mawm."

"Iron Mom?"

She laughed that wild, unfettered laugh of a toddler who just learned what a joke is.

"Yeah! Iron Mom! You made a joke."

The Question

"How old is your daughter?"

"She's two and a half."

"Oh, that's a fun age. Does she have diabetes?"

"No."

"Will she get it, too?"

And this is where I end up tangled in my words and in my emotions. Sometimes I rattle off statistics ("The chances of my daughter developing type 1 are only slightly higher than a non-diabetic mom, while if it were my husband who had diabetes, her chances would be more elevated,"), and sometimes I respond, "No," and roll their question around in my head for a while.

Please don't ask me this question. It hurts more than all the others. I can answer, "Can you eat that?" and "Do you have the 'bad diabetes?'" until my voice is hoarse from answering because it's about me, and I can handle me. But when it comes to my Bird, I don't want to discuss her health. I don't want to talk about anything that could hurt her. My head isn't in the sand, but I thought my heart was walled up tight, to the point where I didn't have a visceral reaction to something as simple as a question.

(It's not walled up at all, though.)

I know why they ask. I have that Thought, too. When people ask this question, my knees go weak while my back muscles tense up, bringing my shoulders back and squared off. "The chances of my daughter getting diabetes are only slightly increased over the chances of anyone else's kid."

What I want to say is, "I love that child with everything I have and even though I know she's okay and even if she ends up with diabetes, she'll still be okay, I don't want to think about her living with a disease. Any disease."

I want people to be aware that I'm already aware of the fact that being a parent means I worry about things I didn't even know existed as potential panic points until two and a half years ago. And I want them to be aware that my child, despite being the daughter of a person with a chronic illness, is still my daughter, and it's hard to think about any potential hardship in her life. We don't want to focus and worry about things that could happen.

Ask me her favorite color. Or ask about her favorite Thomas the Tank Engine train. Ask me what ice cream flavor makes her giggle. Ask me what songs make her dance like a lunatic. Don't ask me about her health. Don't make her feel like she's a ticking time bomb.

We just want to enjoy one another.

Just let us enjoy this.

For Your Blood's Sugar

"I need just a few minutes and then we can definitely go outside."

I took a long draw from the bottle of juice in the fridge (yes, right from the bottle - don't drink the juice at my house unless you want an all-access pass to my germs) and wiped my mouth with my sleeve. My Dexcom was hollering incessantly and it wasn't until I had already popped a glucose tab that I double-checked the beeping against my meter.

"That is a four and a seven. That's four-seven."

"Forty-seven, and mommy needs to take a little break and have some snacks to bring up my blood sugar, okay?"

She nodded, grabbing the Dexcom off of the kitchen table and holding it in her hand. "I watch this while you have a snack."

She pointed to the colors on the Dexcom graph - "White, and then this part is red and it's at the bottom and," "BEEEEEEEEEP!" "Okay, now it beeps again, Mommy." - while I went on auto-pilot, closing the door to the bathroom, making sure the child-safety look on the kitchen sink cabinet was secured, and making sure the step stool was in the cupboard and not out on the floor.

Even though I knew the glucose tabs would hit my system in time, and even though I didn't feel any waves of unconsciousness lapping at the edges of my mind, I wanted to make sure that, if something were to go wrong, my kid was as safe as I could manage.

We went to sit on the floor of her room, and I watched her play as I waited patiently for my blood sugar to come up. She cooked fervently in her kitchen, throwing pieces of plastic food into the red cooking pot and stirring as if her life depended on it. "I'm making cookies," she said as she tossed an artichoke and an ear of corn into the pot. "It's for your bloods sugar."

The Dexcom yowled one more time, reminding me that I wasn't out of the hypoglycemic woods just yet.

"You have some of these cookies and that will stop the beeping, Mom."

"Good goal, kid." I watched her stir in some plastic pears. "Those are cookies, though? You sure about that?"

"Yeah. Cookies."

As the arrow on my Dexcom arched back upward, I tucked into a bowl of Birdy's pseudo-"delicious cookies, mom," for once, not worried about the carb count.

Proof in the Pretend Pudding

Birdy tore by on a scooter and another little kid followed closely with a plastic shopping cart crammed with toy food.

"We're superheroes!!!" she yelled, out of breath as she zipped by.

"I can tell!" I answered, looking up from my papers.

I am the mom at playgroups who spends some of the time staring at an open Word document on my laptop, tapping away on the keys until the letters Centipede themselves around the screen and eventually come to form coherent thoughts. I'm the mom who gets on the trampoline with her kid (and immediately wishes that she didn't, mostly because I spend the whole time panicking about one of us falling off the edge). And I'm the mom who occasionally fumbles through her purse and pulls out a piece of technology and stares at the graph on the screen, or grabs another piece of tech and bleeds with precision on it, or ferrets out a plastic jar and eats several of those ... giant smarties?

I am a mom with type 1 diabetes.

I sometimes wonder how it might look, through the eyes of the other parents and caregivers. Do they think it's gross that I deal with blood at playgroup? Do they notice that I use hand wipes and carefully wipe down anything I've touched after testing my blood sugar, not because I've bled on everything but more because I want to demonstrate my respect for anyone's potential concerns? Do they think I'm a sugar-addict, sometimes popping glucose tabs into my mouth and simultaneously wiping beads of hypoglycemia sweat off my forehead? Do they notice that my outfits always have a small pump bulge and usually some trailing tubing? Do they think it's unfashionable to have glucose tab dust smeared on the front of my shirt?

What's most likely is that they don't notice at all. What feels like a big deal to me at times seems like an unremarkable blip on their overall parenting radar. They probably see another parent, just doing their parenting thing, and are unaware of the small, tangible differences. (I bet they'd notice if I didn't shower, though. That's a hard one to miss.)

"Mom, come make pretend pudding with me! In this little, toy kitchen with these real other kids!"

"Pretend pudding? How can I resist?"

I am a mom with diabetes, not a-bunch-of-diabetes with a side of motherhood. The proof is in the (pretend) pudding.

Put On Your Listening Ears

Our backyard is big and lovely and fenced in on all sides so that when Birdy and I are playing outside, we're both safe from cars and giant woodland creatures (except the ones that can shimmy underneath the fence ... I'm looking at you, groundhog). I don't keep my eyes glued to her while she plays, and we can enjoy the sunshine and the garden without feeling paranoid about passing cars, the kid wandering off, etc.

Which is exactly what sucks about the front yard, because that's the part of the house that the road is closest to. So while I still need to do things in the front yard (getting the mail, tending the front garden, drawing hopscotch in the driveway), I don't do anything of those things without having Birdzone front and center in both my mind and my actual line of sight.

Yesterday evening, Birdy and I were working in the front yard garden (I was clearing out some weeds and she was making houses for worms we discovered underneath a rock), when my Dexcom started wailing from my pocket. In retrospect, I felt a little scrambled, but it wasn't until I heard the low alarm blaring from the Dexcom receiver that the symptoms kicked in fully.

"Hey, your blood sugar is whoa, Mom," Birdy said absently, placing another worm onto a pile of dirt.

"Yeah, we need to go inside and get some snacks, okay? It's important," I replied, looking at the "UNDER 65 MG/DL" warning on the Dexcom screen.

Normally, she listens. Especially when it's about blood sugars, because Chris and I have talked with her a few times about how listening is important, particularly when I tell her my blood sugar is low. But she wanted to stay outside. She liked playing with the worms. She liked being in the dirt and gardening. She didn't want to have to cut playtime short because Mommy needed a few glucose tabs that she should have brought outside with her in the first place.

[*Insert Mom Guilt here.*]

"Nooooo waaaaaaay!!!" she said, flouncing away from me and refusing to turn around.

Under normal circumstances, I would have laughed (because "no way!" is a great response), but I was starting to feel shaky and my brain cells connections felt loose, like thoughts weren't coupling up the right way. We were in the front yard and I knew I needed to gain control of all potentially dangerous situations in a hurry.

"We need. To go. INSIDE right now. My blood sugar is low. This is not a joke." I said.

"No! I don't waaaaaaant to!!"

My blood sugar falls fast. It always has. I don't get the long, lingering slides towards hypoglycemia but instead the quick, breathless plummets. Knowing that I was dropping and watching yet another car drive by our house meant I needed to get control fast and without issue.

Before my body completely caved to the low blood sugar, I scooped up my flailing daughter and walked into the house. She was freaking out and still forcefully asserting her right to "NOOOO!" but I needed sugar more than I needed her to like me.

A few seconds later, we were both safely contained in the kitchen. I had a few glucose tabs and waited for my brain to acknowledge them. Birdy pouted in the corner, staring at her hands and still mumbling "no way."

A few minutes later, I felt more human. "Birds, I'm sorry we had to come inside. But my blood sugar was low and it could have become an emergency. So that's why you needed to put your listening ears on and come inside. I wasn't doing it to be mean; I was doing it to be safe. Does that make sense?"

"Yes."

"I'm sorry we couldn't stay outside. But we can go back out now, okay?"

"Okay. I'm sorry I didn't listen."

"It's okay."

She turned around and pressed her hand into mine. Something wriggled. She smiled.

"I brought a worm inside."

No way.

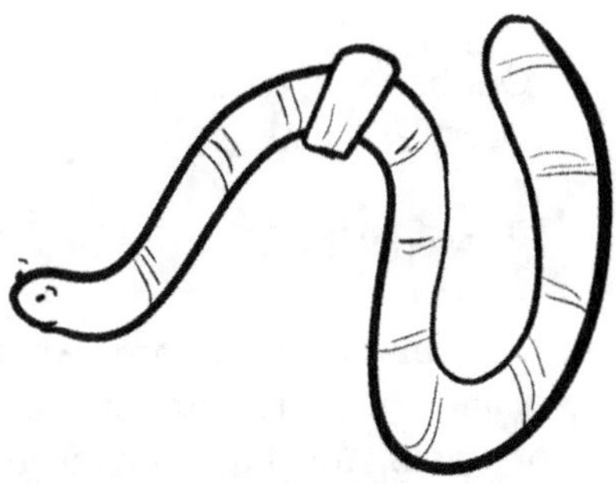

Instead of Making Insulin

"What's insulin?" my daughter asked me as I was buckling her into the car seat.

She knows the word because vials of insulin sit where the butter usually resides in other people's refrigerators.

"Insulin is a hormone that people's pancreases make. It helps make the foods we eat into something our bodies can use for energy. My pancreas doesn't make any insulin, so I put it into my body using my pump or the needles," is my explanation.

"Right. And that's why you have diabetes and dad and I don't," she replies.

"Exactly. My pancreas is lazy sometimes. Instead of making insulin, maybe my pancreas goes to the beach?"

She latched onto this idea immediately. "Yeah! Instead of making insulin, your pancreas goes on a Ferris wheel!"

"Instead of making insulin, my pancreas has an ice cream party!"

"Oooh, oooh! Instead of making insulin, your pancreas goes to the library and listens to story time and then takes out three books!"

"Very specific!"

The game went on for the entire car ride home. "Instead of making insulin, your pancreas writes a letter to Santa!" "Instead of making insulin, my pancreas takes a trip around the moon!" "Instead of making insulin, your pancreas jumps on a trampoline!" "Instead of making insulin, my pancreas grows peanuts on a peanut farm!" "Instead of making insulin, your pancreas hangs out on Sundays with Batman!"

As the car pulled into the driveway, we were giggling madly about the adventures of my under-employed pancreas, outlined in great detail.

"Mom, your pancreas is extremely silly."

"It totally is."

"I wish it made insulin, though," she said, snapping reality back into place in that plain, matter-of-fact way only she can. She gave me a grin that made my heart swell and my pancreas shift uncomfortably in its seat.

"Yep. Me too, love."

Motherhood with Diabetes

"What is that?" my daughter's friend asked me from over her plate of scrambled eggs as I was watching the two kids for the morning.

Before I could answer, my kid piped up, "That's her insulin pump. It has insulin in it."

"Oh," the other three-year-old answered, mouth full of eggs. "What's it for?"

"It has my medicine in it, for diabetes. Remember?" I said, reminding my daughter's friend of conversations we had at the beach over the summer, when she had previously asked me about my insulin pump.

"Yeah. Hey, what's that tunnel?"

Birdy interrupted again: "That's the tubing and it goes into her body and the insulin goes in the tube – insulin comes from a small bottle you cannot touch – and the tube is really squishy and Loopy likes to chase it," and right on cue, the cat came leaping out of nowhere and batted at the pump tubing dangling between my hands as I primed my pump.

Both girls laughed. "LOOPY!!!"

Loopy twirled, chirped, and scampered back into the living room in a flurry of gray fur. The girls resumed breakfast, and I resumed prepping my new infusion set.

"Sometimes my mom has whoa blood sugars but most of the time we just eat the glucose tabs and then it's all better and we go back to playing with the dollhouse," Birdy offered.

"What's a glucose tab?" her friend asked.

"Oh, those are these!!" Birdy leapt down from her chair and ran off to grab one of the blue jars.

"Sometimes mom lets me have a very, very, very small bite. Do you want a very, very, very small bite?"

"YES!"

Which is how my daughter and her friend ended up chasing their scrambled eggs with very, very, very small bites of glucose tabs.

Do You Wish You Didn't Have Diabetes?

"Hang on two more seconds, kiddo. I need to check my blood sugar before we go."

She watches me casually as she slides her arm through the sleeve of her sweatshirt.

"Mom, do you wish you didn't have diabetes?"

She asks me this question all the time now. While diabetes is not a secret in our house, it's not a hot topic of conversation. Instead, she sees what my pump looks like and knows what my Dexcom does, and she likes to push the button on my lancing device to deploy the needle when I need to check. She knows that glucose tabs are for low blood sugars and that I apologize for being unreasonably grouchy when my blood sugar is frustratingly high. A few times she's seen me cry because I was low, but I try to explain to her that it feels bad in the moment but then I feel okay. Most of this becomes threads in the fabric, but lately, she's been asking me that one, specific question on repeat.

"Mom, do you wish you didn't have diabetes?"

My answer is generally the same every time, because I don't want to lie to her. I am not filled with diabetes-loathing, and even though this disease is the single biggest negative issue I deal with every day, I don't feel entirely devoured by it. But I don't like this disease. It's a complicated half-way. There are moments that are compromised, but my life as a whole is not.

"I don't like having diabetes, but I'm fine. I like having you. And having Daddy. And having Looper and Siah Sausage," and then I redirect to something else because I don't want to have long, drawn out discussions with my introspective daughter who has already queried me about how many birthdays people have left.

I think about how diabetes is something normal to her, and always has been. Moms wear insulin pumps, and it furrowed her brow for years that my friends here at home don't have a pump clipped to their hip. Moms carry purses filled with crayons and hand wipes for kids, and then a jar of glucose tabs for when the car is hard to find in the parking lot. Mom's bike basket has a bottle of water and a Dexcom receiver in it. Moms sometimes say, "Let me check my blood sugar first," before going outside to play. This is her normal, too.

"Mom, are you glad I don't have diabetes?"

"I am glad you are exactly who you are. If you ever get diabetes, we'll handle it. When it comes to cookies, we're the toughest," and I breathe out as slowly, slowly, slowly as I can.

A Matter of Apologies

"I was low. I was frustrated because of the low blood sugar. I'm sorry."

"It's okay," and I can tell she means it by the look in her friendly, brown eyes.

I used to be very terrible at saying, "I'm sorry." I would hold on to frustration and anger in a way that was not good for me or anyone around me, making a grudge or the need to feel like I won the disagreement take precedence over a relationship. I'd keep the "I'm sorry" under my tongue because I didn't want to admit that I'd done something that hurt someone's feelings. I felt embarrassed to admit my shortcomings. It felt awkward and bad.

It took a long time for my head to figure out that my heart was better off if I let the sorry fly, but once I came to that realization, I tried to embrace as often as I could. (I also had to work on the "does this interaction make me better or worse as a person?" This is still a work in progress.)

Now I'm less terrible at saying, "I'm sorry," and I feel better for it.

As much as I hate to admit it, my blood sugars are not only influenced by my emotions (stress, anyone?) but they influence my emotions, as well. The way my numbers make me physically feel can cause me to act like a total crumb. It's another reason to be aware of what my blood sugars are, and if I enter the Crumb Zone, apologize for it.

I find myself apologizing to my daughter at times for entirely blood sugar related reasons. Sometimes I snap because I'm taking yet another bolus to correct yet another high and my body is riddled with sugar and rage, and I will be far less than patient with my little one as a result.

Other times I raise my voice because I'm trying to treat a low blood sugar reaction and she's at my elbow asking to [insert rogue request from active 5-year-old here]. Losing my patience during the course of run-of-the-mill parenting is something I am not proud of, but losing my patience because diabetes is leaning on my parenting style is something I want my kid to understand as best she can, because I don't want her ever thinking my seemingly random outbursts are tied to her in any way.

It's a weird balance between feeling like I'm blaming diabetes for my actions and simply explaining my actions. Am I in the Crumb Zone (or Mayor of Crumb City, if you're nasty) because of diabetes? Nope. Diabetes doesn't get credit or get blamed. But sometimes this disease is part of the explanation, and I want my family to have a sense for how, and why, I'm wired a certain way.

There are moments when Birdy assumes my attitude problem is diabetes-related when it's not, and I'm forced to fess up.

"Are you in a bad mood because of a low blood sugar?" my daughter asks, pointedly.

"Not at the moment. Right now, I'm in a bad mood because I just realized I left a banana in the car while I was on my trip last week. And now I'm afraid to open the door and confront the banana stink."

"It's okay," she says. And then adds, "Ew."

The One About Steel Magnolias

I remember sitting down to watch this movie, not knowing how it ended.

"How scary can it be? Julia Roberts has such a big laugh. Mom likes Sally Field. Diabetes in it, too? That's cool. Let's make some popcorn."

record scratch

Narrator's voice: Yeah, that was me, around the age of 10. I didn't know anything about the movie Steel Magnolias that would have given me pause. I knew one of the main characters had type 1 diabetes, and by looking at the cover of the VHS tape, they all looked reasonably smiley and happy, so let's give it a watch.

I didn't know that Steel Magnolias was a true story. I had no idea that a pregnancy with diabetes could take the journey that Shelby's did. I didn't know that it wouldn't be easier
I didn't know diabetes could be that … scary.

Yes, I lived in a bubble. Only a few years into my diabetes diagnosis and barely into the double digits of life, I knew diabetes required attention and discipline and could have some really dark moments but everything would be okay, right? Wouldn't it be okay if I just kept trying?

I don't remember being told that pregnancy would be too hard. I do remember the many people who, upon seeing my pregnant belly in 2010 and in 2016, would look furtively to the side, and then back at me, asking in a low voice "Have you seen Steel Magnolias?"

Yes, I have seen Steel Magnolias. I have seen the wedding colors of blush and bashful and have always wondered where bashful would fall on the pantone palette. I saw them grab Shelby's cheeks with two hands in the hair salon, forcing the glass of juice to her mouth, Clairee leaning in to offer, "She's a diabetic." I watched M'Lynn lose the chance to take a whack at Ouiser.

I cried at this movie. A lot. For a dozen different reasons, thinking about my own mother, my own children, my own fears, and my own disease. My own frailties. My own strength. (I also cried because I'm a movie crier. Coffee commercial crier, too. I am often dehydrated.)

But "I would rather have 30 minutes of wonderful than a lifetime of nothing special."

Steel Magnolias came out in 1989, three years after my diagnosis. At the time, it colored my views of diabetes with a blush and bashful brush, painting the possibilities of parenthood with hesitation and concern. Even when I had more hope and had seen evidence of healthy pregnancies with diabetes, I would push the thoughts of M'Lynn out of my mind and jokingly tell friends, "Not Shelby," when they asked what names we had picked out for my daughter. Shelby's story was a true story, but it was a story from 30 years ago, and didn't define every diabetic's experience with pregnancy, or a wedding, or even the hairdresser. I think about that in the context of all the diabetes stories on social media, acknowledging how each story is unique and diverse within this shared disease experience.

Steel Magnolias was often held up to me as something to fear, but I found it weirdly inspirational. It was her real life. And I loved Shelby's story because it wasn't about diabetes, necessarily. It was about those women, and their friendships, and about family. It was about living beyond a diabetes diagnosis.

I wanted that. I want that.

And I look at my kids, one about to turn 8 and the other fast approaching two, and know that every worry, every moment of concern has been worth it. They have provided more than 30 minutes of wonderful. They've given me a lifetime of something special.

Learning Empathy

"Pump! Pump, pump, pump! Pump, where are you?"

It's his siren call, yelled at full volume as my toddler forages around in my top trying to find my insulin pump. "Oh hi, pump! One … two … three!" and the buttons are pressed and the beeps are beeped and I'm constantly checking to make sure he hasn't given me a bolus.

I told him the other day that there's "insulin" in my pump, which made him nod sagely. "Insuwin," he replied, putting his finger deftly into my ear.

Parenting with diabetes is a trip. It's this weird dance of making sure the mischief of my diabetes is managed well enough so that I can play with my kids without tipping over. The majority of the time, diabetes isn't a parenting hurdle, but there are plenty of moments when I trip over my blood sugars. Especially now, with the hard-earned circus of two kids.

In my house, I have an eight-year-old and an almost-two-year-old. Both kids are mobile, both kids talk, and both kids have opinions and preferences that don't always line up with one another. Their gentle ribbons of chaos wind around the unpredictable pole of diabetes nonsense and we become this mixed metaphor of a maypole.

I'm trying to raise my kids while wrangling diabetes, and I'm not great at doing both all the time. We make it sort of work (thankfully they get along really well at the moment), but these days, the activity level is usually amped to 11 because whatever we're doing always includes movement. As a result, my lows have been on the unpredictable side because I can't predict if the little Guy will want to sit still and read a book or if he wants to tear down the aisles of the library touching all the books and asking to listen to The Pancake Song on repeat.

My son is learning about diabetes similarly to how I taught my daughter – repeated, gentle exposure to the visible management bits. One of my son's first words was "pump," and it remains the best tool I have in my parenting arsenal to keep him from rolling off the diaper changing table.

He's also recently learned the word "Dexcom," as a result of the mantra, "Careful – Mommy's Dexcom is right there" as he climbs all over my legs and threatens to pull off my sensors. This morning, there was a mostly-consumed juice box on my bathroom counter that my son sauntered in, grabbed, and finished off before I could stop him.

"Mommy's juice!"

He was delighted by the reward at the end of this scavenger hunt of maternal hypoglycemia.

Explaining to him that a symptom of low blood sugar might be his mom bursting frustratedly into tears will take some time. Or that a sustained high blood sugar might make me exhausted, and short-tempered. Or that diabetes has a number of IFs, ANDs, and BUT ...s to it. My daughter only recently began to understand that concept. The nuances of diabetes take some time for kids to understand.

... takes a long time for adults to understand, too.

Explaining diabetes to my kids is a lifelong journey. They'll grow up thinking that diabetes is normal, that it's something mom handles and needs help with here and there but isn't classified as "a huge deal" because at the moment, the chaos is controlled.

And that's where my hard work and hope intersect: I hope diabetes is always a small deal, with most of the work and responsibility on my plate, without too many other health issues in play. I am motivated to continue to try because I want diabetes to remain small. And I hope that growing up with a mother who has health concerns will teach my children something good, you know?

It starts with stealing their fruit snacks, but my hope is that it becomes patience, empathy, and compassion.

Thoughts on Being a Mom with Type 1 Diabetes

Being a mom with type 1 diabetes isn't something I think about often because, on the average, run-of-the-mill day, diabetes doesn't influence the way I mom. (And as the mother of two very active kids, "to mom" is definitely a verb. We don't sit still very often.) Being pregnant with type 1 diabetes was very intense and at times dominated that experience, but after the kids were born, diabetes came off the front burner and went back to being that awkward pot on the back.

The small, almost unseen details are where diabetes affects my parenting now.

My son is not yet three, but he's starting to notice some things are different about his mom's body than other moms' bodies. Like when I hold him and he uses the pump infusion site on the back of my arm like a rock wall crimp (and I almost immediately say, "Don't pull Mom's pump off ... don't ... pull ... it ...").

"That's MOMMY's juice, for bwoodsugars," my toddler says, pointing to the juice box on the bedside table. "Don't touch it," he says again, pointing to his own chest.

Or when my pump alarms and he immediately bursts into his own parroting back of the tune.

"You pump is beeping. You beeping, Mom. You have a beeps."

I have many a beeps.

My daughter is older, newly-minted nine-year-old, and knows the difference between type 1 and type 2 diabetes. She is quick to educate people who need more information to understand both kinds.

Birdy also did a presentation at school about Frederick Banting, where she talked about the discovery of insulin, the research roles that dogs played, and the Flame of Hope in London, Ontario. "It was lit in honor of people with diabetes, and the team that discovers the cure will be flown out to extinguish the flame." She paused. "I hope that happens soon, Mom."

I hope so, too.

My kids know their mom has some robot parts and an affinity for fruit snacks whilst sweaty and shaking, but I hope that diabetes lives on the surface level for them.

The places where diabetes lurks the darkest and deepest, though, is something you can't see at all. It's the swirling synapses of my brain, wondering if diabetes will only affect my body or if it will ever affect my children's physical forms. I am asked if they have diabetes, too at every single conference I have spoken at since the birth of my daughter. My response, so far, is always the same: "No, they don't." And then there's this weird pause, where the person asking leans in a little bit, waiting for more of a response.

But I don't have more to say. They don't have diabetes. They know what diabetes is (or are learning). We're just figuring parenting/kidding out as we go, making some of our strategies up on the fly. If a diagnosis hits us, we'll wrangle it the best we can. Just like we'll handle anything else that comes our way.

I can't really imagine what it's like to be a mom who doesn't have diabetes. What do you mean, you don't always have snacks on you? What do you mean, kids asking for an extra sippy cup doesn't make your stomach drop, too? What do you mean, you have butter in your butter compartment? Ha! That's not what that compartment is for!

My ability to parent is not diminished by diabetes. My pancreas is a bit of a garbage can but the rest of me can still run headlong into parenting with all the love and care my kids deserve.

(there's a bit more ...)

Afterword

That's it. These essays are selections from fourteen years of writing SixUntilMe.com, and they are the ones that will stand as an archive of my experience as a diabetes blogger.

What a weird gig, by the way. Writing online about a health condition – that's a hobby I didn't see coming. It makes sense, though. I always felt as though diabetes was a serious health condition but really easy to be subtle about, leaving very little about diabetes detectable to people outside of the experience. It's easy to hide. It's easy to leave undisclosed.

Until there's a moment when you need someone to know. Maybe because of a low blood sugar, or some other diabetes-related emergency. Or maybe because you need to talk about it, to process the emotions of it – that's just as much a "need someone to know" moment as any other. After decades with diabetes, I now realize that being open about diabetes helps me live better with it.

Writing about diabetes has really helped me, in a dozen different ways, for a dozen different reasons. Being tuned in to the emotional experience of diabetes helps me understand myself as a human, and helps me achieve my goal of being a healthy, old person someday.

I look forward to the honor of being an ancient, wizened woman, sitting comfortably in a chair made of pixels and telling my robot great-grandchildren about how I used to take insulin with needles but still traveled the world and created a life worth writing down with my stubborn little pancreas in tow.

Glossary of People and Frequently Used Terms

For friends who haven't read SixUntilMe.com before, here's a starter glossary of some of the people and terms mentioned in these essays:

Abby the Cat: an enormous calico cat we lost in 2012; she's first because this is an alphabetical list

Balancing Diabetes: the title of my first book, published in 2014; this title was created by the publisher, for sure, because I would never claim to know how to balance diabetes

Birdy: my daughter, also known as Birdzone, Birds, or Bsparl

Chris: my husband; he's the best husband, the best dad, and also an excellent human

CGM: continuous glucose monitor; I have been wearing different iterations of the Dexcom CGM since 2006

DOC (Diabetes Online Community): the diabetes community online existed for decades before I started writing my blog, living in message boards and Usenet groups and in websites established when I was very young. When I became aware of it, and subsequently joined it, blogs and social media sites like Twitter became where many of my community touchpoints lived. Around the time when blogging became popular, the acronym "D.O.C." became shorthand for the 'diabetes online community.'

The Little Guy: my son (he was born shortly before I stopped blogging, so he didn't get an internet moniker that stuck as squarely as his sister's)

Loki: tabby cat who gained plenty of weight during the pandemic and is now a round mound of lazy

Loopy: she's fluffy, she's gray, and at the time of publication, she's still alive; also a cat

Pump: earliest essays mention a Medtronic 512 insulin pump, then I moved on to an Animas Ping, and finally a Tandem t:slim; please see relevant disclosures

Prussia the Cat: a tabby cat, also known as PTC, who passed away in 2013

PWD: short for "people with diabetes"

Rage Bolus: "The act of taking an aggressive correction dose of insulin after experiencing prolonged and frustrating high blood sugar. Often results in a hypoglycemic event;" a term I coined in 2005 and is also the title of my diabetes poetry book (2021)

Rhode Island: the state we live in, often questioned to be "Long Island?" by people who live in the United States who still don't know that Rhode Island is a STATE for crying out loud

Siah Sausage: a fat gray cat who hated everyone who didn't live in our house; passed away in 2016

Six Until Me: the diabetes-centric blog I started in May of 2005; the blog name was an attempt at a poetic interpretation of when diabetes symptoms first cropped up in my timeline; you can find that essay, She Still Smiles, on the next ... page ... turn it ... now!

She Still Smiles

It was six years, until me.

I didn't know her before my arrival, but from what I hear, she was a good kid. Running all over the place. Devouring every book she could find. This kid even read in the shower when she was that small. Bloated, damp books strewn about the bathroom. She tortured her sister relentlessly. She tried to play the games her older brother taught her.

She smiled a lot. And laughed out loud.

I'm not sure when I was called out to stay with her, but I've been told it was when she was sick as a little kid on her sixth birthday.

She had a fever that lasted for days. Lethargic little thing, under the careful watch of her ever-vigilant mother. I remember visiting her then, settling gently into her tiny body and making it my home. No one knew I was there. They wouldn't know for six more months.

Six months until me.

I didn't mean to embarrass her. But she started to wet the bed after I arrived. Just over six years old and wetting the bed again. She also had a ratty little pillow she needed to cuddle with when she fell asleep. I made her blood sugar so high in the middle of the night that she couldn't help it: she would wet the bed. And nothing, not the encouragement of her parents, the dreaded pee alarm, or the shame she felt, could make her stop.

She quit that cuddle pillow cold turkey. "If I can't stop wetting the bed, then I'm going to stop this!" I felt bad. I had no intention of making her feel so frustrated.

She doesn't remember much of her own diagnosis, but I do. I remember when they found me. I remember when she peed in the cup at the doctor's office before she started second grade and they detected the ketones. They called her parents. Her mom and dad brought her in for follow up bloodwork. And then they found me. September 1986.

She didn't cry much. Her mom and dad brought her to the hospital, where she stayed for two weeks. Her parents bought her a stuffed Kitty that she toted around everywhere... the doctors became used to her little face and the presence of the stuffed animal. She said that Kitty was diabetic, too, and both Kerri and Kitty received injections. The fabric of the animal became a little stained from injecting saline, but it made her smile again. She didn't feel alone.

And she grew up. Even though I was there. She competed in spelling bees. She tap-danced for 15 years. She played soccer, albeit badly. (But I had nothing to do with that.) She kissed a boy. She drove her car. She battled with her parents and confided in her friends. She wrote stories. She keeps a journal, still. She went to college. She moved out on her own. She succeeded. She failed. She adopted too many cats. She fell in love. She dreamed. And then she fell in love again.

She had six years, until me. People thought I would change her life, make her sad. Make her sick. Make her angry.

But instead, I've made her strong. I've made her fearless. And I've made her appreciate everything she has, everything she fights for. She hasn't let me make her choices. She refuses to let me own her. She controls me. When she is in her last moments, whether sixty years from now or today, she will know, with certainty, that she has Lived.

Really lived.

She still smiles a lot. And laughs out loud.

Disclosures

From 2010 – 2016, I had a sponsorship agreement with Animas Corporation, during which time I was compensated as a spokesperson and received pump supplies as part of my compensation.

From 2016 to the time of this publication (September 2022), I have a sponsorship contract with Tandem Diabetes Care. You can read details of that agreement here:

kerrisparling.com/disclosures

Please keep these agreements in mind when reading about my experiences with aforementioned insulin pumps.

Acknowledgements

Thank you to my family and friends for being okay with years of, "I just need to hit publish on this post!" and for letting me share some of our family's story on the Internet. Without the steadfast support of my husband, my children, and my family, I would have never had the courage to share my story with the world wide web. Through their encouragement, I found my voice, and my community.

Chris, Ava, and Jake - I love you with my whole heart.

Thank you to my parents and siblings for keeping the focus off "diabetes" and instead keeping the focus on the "life with" part.

Thank you to all the people who have been part of my diabetes family for years. To the first fellow diabetes blogger I found, Scott Johnson, to Amy Tenderich, and then Nicole, Tek, Dee, Shannon, Juilia, and Violet. Those first few connections in the DOC were everything to me.

To you, the people who have been reading SixUntilMe.com since the beginning – thank you. And thank you to those who have stumbled into or sought out this book. Thank you for giving me purpose in this way. Thank you for making time to be part of my life. Thank you for letting me be part of yours. And thank you for your continued support in whatever's next.

To say "I love you" wouldn't feel wrong.

So, I love you.

Thanks for every last bit of all of this.

ABOUT THE AUTHOR

Kerri Sparling is a writer, poet, and speaker who has dedicated her life to amplifying the patient narrative. Since 2005, she has been a leading voice in the patient advocacy space, sharing her personal story of over 36 years with type 1 diabetes while helping share stories from others in the patient community. Kerri has worked to bolster the influence of patient stories in the healthcare space, from academic journals to keynote presentations around the world.

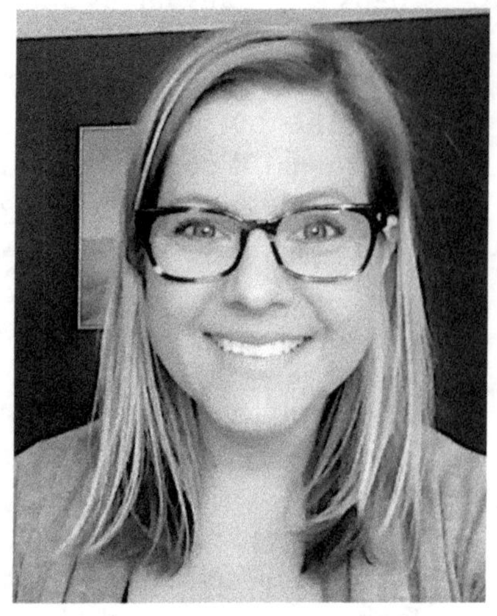

She is best known for her work as a patient storyteller at SixUntilMe.com, and is the author of *Balancing Diabetes* (2014), *Rage Bolus* (2021), and *Six Until Me* (2022). You can keep up with Kerri's latest works at KerriSparling.com

Kerri lives in Rhode Island with her husband and children.

To connect with Kerri, you can email her at kerri (at) kerrisparling (dot) com.

9 798833 368268